D0515128

Toilet training for
Individuals with Autism or other Developmental Issues

A Comprehensive Guide for
Parents & Teachers

MARIA WHEELER

Hay Library
Western Wyoming Community College

Toilet Training

All marketing and publishing rights guaranteed to and reserved by

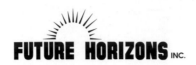

FUTURE HORIZONS INC.

721 W. Abram Street
Arlington, Texas 76013
800-489-0727
817-277-0727
817-277-2270 (fax)
E-mail: info@FHautism.com
www.FHautism.com

© Copyright 2007, Maria Wheeler, M.Ed.

All rights reserved.

Printed in Canada.

No part of this book may be reproduced in any manner whatsoever
without written permission of Future Horizons, Inc., except in the case of brief
quotations embodied in reviews.

ISBN: 1-932565-49-3
ISBN 13: 978-1932565-49-2

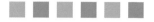

This book is dedicated to all of the children, adults, families, and educators who gave me the privilege of viewing autism from their own unique viewpoints. Thank you for giving me the perspective, understanding, and experience to make a real difference. Your generosity, shown through sharing ideas, frustrations, successes, and life experience, adds quality and promise to the lives of others.

Acknowledgments

I wish to express my gratitude to Chris, Sarah, Josh, and the other children who taught me about the realities of toilet training and provided my earliest challenging experiences—which resulted in adult tears, children's tantrums and hours spent cleaning. These children's needs for social acceptance and independence provided me with the motivation to learn more about this topic through extensive research and persistent exploration of interventions that remove barriers to success and promote mastery of this basic skill. Armed with this new knowledge, our early frustration quickly grew into the satisfaction of accomplishment and autonomy.

I wish to thank Wayne Gilpin and Future Horizons, Inc. for expert advice and assistance with this endeavor.

A special thank you is extended to Jennifer Gilpin for suggesting the idea to write this book.

Table of Contents

Foreword

Carol S. Kranowitz, M.A.

There are three things you cannot make another person do: sleep, eat, and poop. Since time began, every child has experimented with controlling his own body. While the typically-developing child usually learns to regulate these basic functions, individuals with autism may have a harder time getting in sync. For them, toilet training can be extraordinarily challenging.

Annie, a seven-year-old with autism, has learned to have a bowel movement in the toilet after breakfast. She can wipe her bottom, pull up her underpants, and wash and dry her hands. But she refuses to flush. Why? Because, she cries, "Annie made it!" Flushing would mean throwing away a precious product of her own body.

Bobby, a sixth-grader with autism, panics about using the bathroom at school. Why? Because the acoustically harsh sounds of flushing toilets and gushing faucets in the boys' room overload his sensitive auditory system. He would rather try to "hold it" than enter that torture chamber.

Curtis, a teenager with Asperger's Syndrome, defecates in his pants instead of using the bathroom at his learning center. Why? Because he has dyspraxia, a sensory-based motor disorder. He cannot come up with the idea of unbuttoning and unzipping his pants, how to motor plan these tasks, and how to carry out the plan. Easily discouraged by such a complex sequence of actions, he does not even try.

Donald, an autistic young man in his twenties, prefers diapers. Why? Because the weight and pressure of a diaper loaded with his own waste is tactilely soothing on his skin.

All individuals with autism are unique, and the reasons for their toileting problems are varied. One reason may be misunderstanding, like little Annie who believes she may flush away a part of herself. Other reasons may be that the person gets distracted, or is unaware that it is time to have a bowel movement, or becomes upset when making a mess, or has a meltdown when being scolded for not cooperating.

Often, an underlying and very common reason for toileting problems is difficulty in processing sensory messages. This problem, called Sensory Processing Disorder (SPD), afflicts almost all people with ASD.

How does SPD play out when it comes to toileting?

Some individuals may be over-responsive to sensations. The noise in the bathroom is overwhelming, or the feeling of the toilet seat against their skin is uncomfortable, or perching on the seat with their feet off the ground makes them fear they will fall in. These sensory avoiders withdraw from sensations and situations that they cannot interpret effectively.

Some individuals are under-responsive to sensations. They may lack the body awareness to know that they need to eliminate. They don't notice that their underpants are full, that their clothes are wet, or that they smell bad. These sensory disregarders ignore important sensations.

Some individuals are sensory seekers. Warm, squishy fecal matter may be comforting to "wear" or to sit on. Smearing it with their hands may be a sensory pleasure and make them feel more alert. These sensory cravers go for stimulation that may not be socially acceptable.

Some individuals have difficulty discriminating among sensory stimuli. They may not distinguish between "empty" and "almost empty," and may jump off the toilet before completing a bowel movement. These sensory jumblers are unable to tell one sensation from another.

Some individuals have a sensory-based motor disorder. One of these is a postural disorder, causing difficulty getting into and maintaining a stable position. It is hard for these sensory slumpers to hold on and stay put. Another sensory-based motor disorder is dyspraxia, a problem illustrated in the above example by Curtis, who is a sensory fumbler.

Maria Wheeler, a wise and compassionate behavior analyst, understands sensory processing difficulties as well as a myriad of other differences that cause toileting problems. In this unique book, she explains all these problems, be they sensory, cognitive, emotional, developmental, or communicative. She presents sensible, doable suggestions to parents, teachers, and caregivers struggling to help people with autism master toileting skills. Her sound advice includes using a person's preference for ritual to help him get the job done, or playing classical music and providing a tabletop with calming toys to make sitting on the toilet a pleasant experience. She offers many case examples to illustrate successes when caregivers observe the person's behavior, realize that behavior means something, and find a solution.

Many thanks to Maria for writing a book about a topic that just won't go away. Someone had to do it, and she has done it splendidly!

—Carol S. Kranowitz, M.A.
Author, *The Out-of-Sync Child*

CHAPTER 1

The Importance of Toilet Training

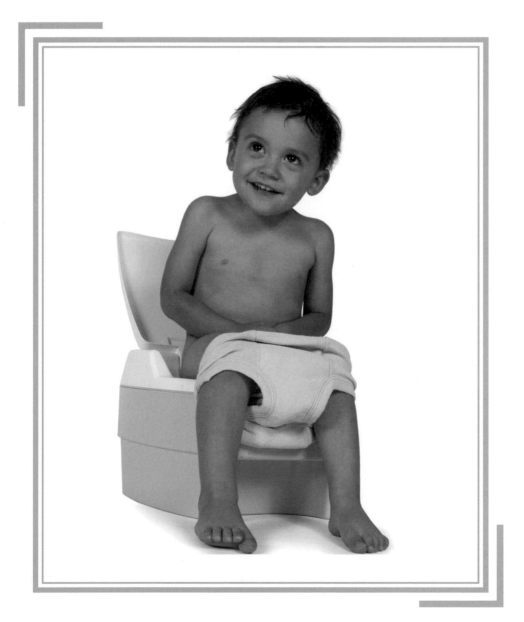

One of the most important skills a person will ever learn is how to use the toilet successfully and independently. Wetting and soiling clothing results in significant amounts of time, energy, and resources being devoted to an individual's personal care needs. Wet or soiled clothing or poor toileting hygiene can also significantly interfere with social acceptance. Some maladaptive behaviors associated with a lack of acceptable toileting skills can present health risks to the individual and care providers. Persons with autism have been reported by researchers to be the most difficult population to toilet train. Many techniques used to toilet train typical children are not sufficient when used to teach toileting skills to persons with autism. There are, however, strategies that have been demonstrated to be effective when teaching toileting skills.

Characteristics of Autism that Influence Toilet Training

Every individual is unique. However, there are particular characteristics associated with autism that impact behavior. These factors have a significant impact on both the successes and challenges you will experience when toilet training. To be successful in one's training efforts, it is essential that the characteristics and needs unique to the individual be considered when planning interventions.

Characteristics to be addressed when planning intervention include:

- Communication needs
- Literal communication
- Sensory awareness
- Sensitivity to stimulation
- Preference for routine or ritual
- Motor planning difficulties
- Limited imitation
- Sequential learning
- Increased levels of anxiety
- Difficulty adjusting behaviors to fit new situations

Communication plays a major role in the toilet training process when an individual relies on caretakers to assist with accessing facilities. Additionally, effective communication must take place in order to teach someone the steps involved in toileting. When planning interventions, keep in mind the tendency for persons with autism to interpret language in a very literal and concrete manner.

Sensory issues also affect responses to toilet training. The degree of awareness of one's own bodily changes related to elimination, sensitivity to tactile stimulation from clothing, and environmental stimulation in the bathroom, all influence the effectiveness of toilet training.

Preferences for routine and ritual can be used as strengths to build upon, turning toileting into a regular routine. Difficulty adjusting behaviors to fit new situations, such as using a different toilet in a new environment, can often be remedied by creating rituals that serve as a bridge between the old routine and new situations. Also, these routines and rituals can be used to present toileting skills as a sequence of steps to provide the necessary sequential learning.

Learning through imitation has significant limits; however, imitation can be a powerful strategy for teaching new skills or behaviors. Remember, imitation of incorrect behaviors can be learned as easily as acceptable skills. When using any form of imitation, rely on effective communication strategies to direct attention to the specific behaviors to imitate. Do not risk leaving this to chance. If attention is sporadic or focused on irrelevant details, the wrong sequence of steps will be learned.

Success with toileting can also be influenced by motor planning difficulties. When an individual experiences problems planning and producing the physical movements required to perform a particular behavior, accessing and using the toilet unassisted can become an overwhelming challenge. It is not uncommon for the person to know what he is supposed to do, but not be able to begin the physical movements needed to execute the task. This may occur consistently or sporadically.

All of the characteristics described can result in increased levels of anxiety, frustration and confusion related to toilet training. These feelings are often expressed in the form of misbehaviors that appear to be resistance to using the toilet or remaining continent. Careful analysis of these characteristics plays an integral role in successfully teaching toileting.

Impact on Home, Family, and Community

The issue of toilet training impacts the home, family, and community in numerous ways. Various families, home situations, and community environments are affected differently. Needs and responses range from a child flushing the toilet several times to adolescents or adults whose independence, jobs, and social lives are threatened by incontinence or poor toileting hygiene. Some families find it easier to leave children in diapers and not address the toileting issue at all. Other families experience extensive anxiety and frustration in their efforts to toilet train their loved one who has autism. Families caring for persons who are not toilet trained experience very high demands on their time, energy, and finances.

In some families, siblings or others may feel embarrassed when a family member is incontinent. The likelihood of this becoming a significant factor often increases when the incontinent family member is older and readily accesses environments outside of the home. The additional attention needed by a person who is not toilet trained or who is learning to use the toilet can result in jealousy from siblings or other family members. These feelings may be expressed through anger, resentment, guilt, or various behavior problems.

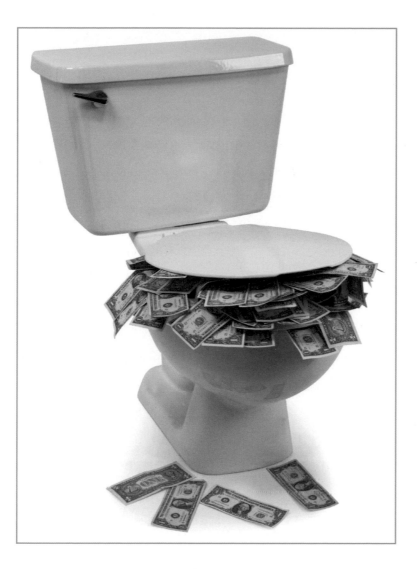

Family finances can easily be consumed by purchasing diapers, clothing, or other materials and equipment needed when a family member has not learned to use the toilet. This may result in resentment if purchases of other desired items are limited because money is being spent on resources for the individual with autism. Additionally, meeting the needs of someone who is not toilet trained can be physically demanding, since lifting or other physical activity is required repeatedly throughout each day. Parents may also question their parenting skills when attempted toilet training techniques are unsuccessful.

When a family member with autism is not toilet trained:

- Recognize the impact on your family and resources.
- Access available resources such as Medicaid or public school noneducational monies to assist in offsetting costs of diapers, equipment, respite care, etc.
- Determine if the person is ready for toilet training.
- Recognize that time and effort invested in effective toilet training is temporary, with demands decreasing significantly when training is complete.
- Realize the long-term impact of toilet training on the person's independence and social acceptance.
- Realize the long-term impact of toilet training on the family's independence, resources, interactions and social acceptance.
- Set aside specific amounts of dedicated time for other family members who may feel deprived of attention.
- Use stress management techniques to decrease the negative effects of extra demands on time and energy.

Impact on School and Learning

Just as it is in the home, toilet training can be physically and emotionally demanding in the school setting. Teachers can experience stress and frustration when toilet training techniques are ineffective, or when regression occurs, and then confidence in teaching skills may be jeopardized. Students may successfully use the toilet at home, but not at school, or vice versa. Some teachers may feel that toilet training is a home responsibility and should not be addressed at school. These situations can lead to resentment or other negative feelings between the school and home.

CASE EXAMPLE

Tommy was five years old. He was not toilet trained. He enjoyed books, TV, movies, and outings to local fast food restaurants and discount stores. Mrs. Jordan had tried to toilet train Tommy when he was four years old, but he resisted being placed on the toilet. Rather than battle with him over toileting issues, Mrs. Jordan decided it was simply easier to keep Tommy in diapers. He stayed dry at school, usually wearing training pants. Mrs. Jordan thought Tommy would eventually decide to use the toilet at home, since he was successfully using the toilet at school. During a parent conference, Tommy's teacher explained to Mrs. Jordan the importance of teaching him to use the toilet at home. She explained he was old enough that wearing a diaper would begin to interfere with his social acceptance and inclusion in community activities. With the teacher's help, Mrs. Jordan learned to use the same toileting routines and picture cues that Tommy used at school. He responded to these supports and was soon using the toilet at home. Mrs. Jordan also took steps to maintain her family's well being while toilet training her son. Since the initial training required that Tommy have her close attention, Mrs. Jordan set aside extra story time for her three-year-old daughter following each toileting session. She also set aside a fifteen-minute relaxation break for herself every evening, after putting the children to bed.

Additionally, the school environment may not be conducive to teaching toileting skills. School restrooms can be large, loud, cold, and frightening in comparision to home bathrooms. Co-workers, supervisors, and support staff may not understand or agree with the teacher's efforts at toilet training, leading the teacher to experience feelings of isolation and rejection by her peers.

When addressing toilet training issues at school:

- Parents and educators need to work together as a team, with student continence throughout each day being their team's goal.
- Parents and educators need to share with one another specific observations and techniques that work in their individual situations and experiences.
- Parents and educators need to support one another's efforts by communicating and providing for various materials and equipment needed for toilet training, such as diapers, extra clothes, potty seats, etc.
- Parents and educators need to support one another's efforts by promptly communicating information that may affect toileting behavior, such as unusual foods ingested or medications given.
- Administrators need to support their teachers' efforts to toilet train students by promptly addressing equipment or other needs involving school resources that present barriers to training.

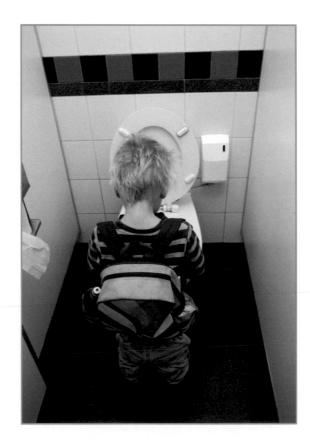

CAUTION !!!

- Avoid blaming or becoming angry with the parent or teacher when toilet training techniques are ineffective. This is the time when it is most important to work together and explore other options for intervention.

- Avoid becoming angry when parents or teachers are overwhelmed with daily demands and forget to send diapers, clothing, other materials, or communications. Always have a back-up plan for such days so minor incidents do not become major obstacles or setbacks.

- Avoid giving up when parent and teacher sources do not result in progress. This is the time when accessing outside assistance is highly indicated. Outside assistance can be accessed from a variety of sources, including books, journal articles, internet information, support groups, other parents or teachers, special education support services, and professionals in the private sector. Carefully evaluate any interventions, including their appropriateness for your individual situation and student, before implementing.

Impact on Social Relationships

Social relationships of both the person with autism and the family can be limited by poor toileting skills. This becomes a greater factor as the individual grows older. Families may become isolated from friends and social contacts because others tend to avoid interaction due to excessive demands on the family's time or the incontinent person's offensive hygiene. Individuals who use effective communication and social skills may continue to have a high rate of negative social experiences if their hygiene skills are offensive. Teaching the basic toileting and hygiene skills needed for social acceptance is an integral part of social skills training and becomes a higher priority with each passing year. The lack of independent toileting skills can severely inhibit an individual's inclusion in school- and community-based activities. Without adequate preparation or planning for toileting needs, situations intended to be socially enhancing can actually subject individuals to ridicule, rejection, or harassment by the persons from whom acceptance and interaction is desired.

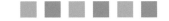

CHAPTER 2

Determining Readiness

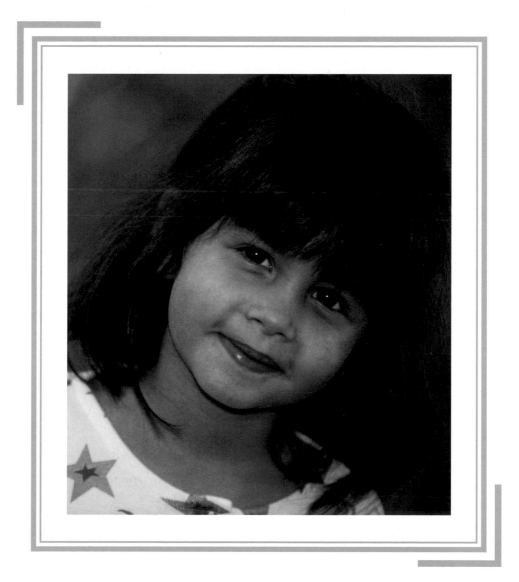

Deciding when a child is ready to begin toilet training can be challenging, especially when the child is two to five years of age and the social impact of being incontinent is minimal. The chronological age of a child, based on actual birthdate, is an important consideration when determining readiness for toilet training. Such training should not begin before eighteen months of age. However, once a person is beyond four years old, toilet training usually should become a priority. Most children need to be continent or be exposed to habit training, as described in Chapter 5, before they are five to six years old.

Chronological vs. Mental Age

Some caretakers are hesitant to begin toilet training individuals who function as if they were four years of age or younger, even when their chronological age is much greater. A person's mental age is an important consideration when deciding if training is appropriate. Mental age is determined by examining an individual's performance levels, as opposed to his or her chronological age. Some persons with autism have a mental age that is different from their chronological age. A person whose mental age is lower than two years may not be a good candidate for toilet training.

Awareness Level

However, all factors influencing the entire set of behaviors required for successful toileting need to be considered when determining readiness. One important consideration is the level of awareness the person has regarding elimination-related issues. It is important to realize that direct awareness or interest is not always obvious in a person with autism. Awareness may be indirectly demonstrated by slight or significant changes in behavior when exposed to particular activities, places, or objects.

Questions to ask when determining awareness regarding elimination-related issues include:

- Does the person act differently or seem to notice when diapers or clothing are wet or soiled?
- Is there any interest or difference in behavior related to the bathroom, toilet, handwashing, dressing, undressing or other related tasks?
- Has any interest or change in behavior been shown in response to seeing other people involved in activities or with objects related to toileting?

Answering "yes" to any of these questions may indicate an appropriate level of awareness for initiating toilet training.

Physiological Factors

Various physiological factors affect readiness for toilet training. Closely related to awareness is the issue of whether the individual is able to remain dry and unsoiled for one to two hours at a time. Another similar measure is whether the person can remain dry and unsoiled during naps. These are sometimes considered to be indications of a person's physical capacity for temporarily retaining bodily wastes in order to remain continent. One additional indicator of physical readiness for bowel training is regular bowel movements and no soiling during sleep.

CAUTION !!!

Avoid postponing toilet training when an individual shows other signs of readiness, but does not remain dry and unsoiled for one to two hour periods or during naps. For persons who eliminate several times per hour due to constant intake of food or drink, consider proceeding with training that includes incorporating scheduled intake of food and drink. For individuals who do not totally void or evacuate when eliminating, include techniques that assist them with fully emptying the bladder and colon while on the toilet. Such techniques are discussed in Chapter 6.

Other Readiness Indicators

A few miscellaneous skills essential for toilet training include:

- The physical ability to sit and hold one's body in a basically upright position
- Basic cooperation with undressing related to toileting, in order to minimize agitation immediately prior to attempting to eliminate
- Freedom from medical conditions that contraindicate participation in a toileting program

CASE EXAMPLE

Sarah was four years old. She enjoyed sipping juice and water throughout most of the day. Mom had to change her diapers frequently, sometimes more than two times per hour. The doctor said nothing was physically wrong with her. Mom started regulating her fluid intake by providing a glass of juice or water every two hours, then putting it away after ten minutes. Sarah began voiding on a predictable schedule and was able to start a toilet training program that was successful.

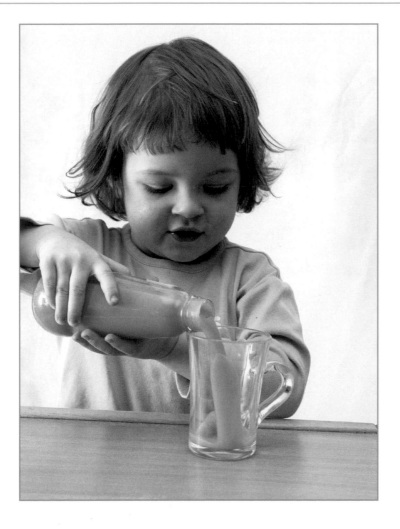

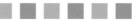

CHAPTER 3

Developing a Toileting Routine

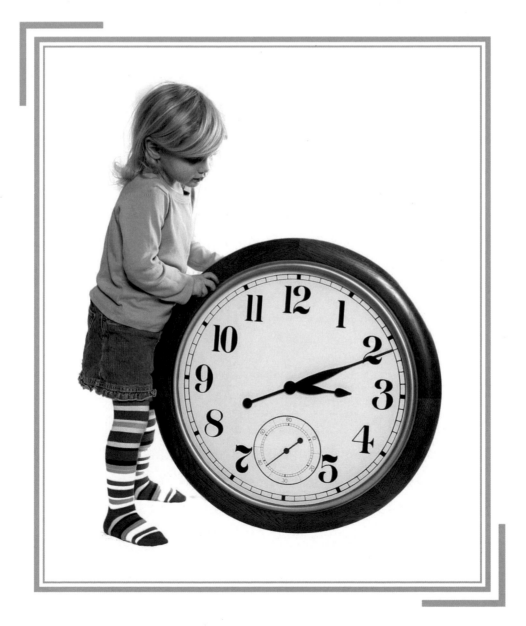

Many persons with autism have a strong preference for routines and rituals. Building on this intense desire for predictability provides one of the most powerful strategies that leads to successful toilet training. Teach using the toilet as an entire routine involving preparation and activities needed for completion, rather than simply teaching the task of sitting on the commode. Approach the toilet training as a whole routine of sequenced behaviors, instead of focusing on simple bladder and bowel control.

Developing Toileting Schedules

View the following as part of the entire toileting routine:

- Follow a visual schedule for eating foods and drinking fluids during toilet training to enhance regular elimination.
- Identify appropriate times for toileting and include those times in the visual schedule.
- Check the schedule, enter the bathroom, undress, sit on the commode, wipe, flush, dress, wash and dry hands, and return to check the next scheduled activity.

Developing and consistently following regularly scheduled times for accessing the toilet significantly increases the effectiveness of training. In order to develop a schedule, careful observation of the individual's current elimination habits is needed. Recording the information observed, such as writing on a chart the time of day when the person voids or has a bowel movement, allows for accuracy and more effective planning. Unpredictable or irregular elimination habits indicate a greater need for charting the information in order to develop a reasonable schedule that can be followed consistently. Begin by developing a schedule for waking hours only. Nighttime training should only be considered after the person develops a reasonable degree of independence with daytime toileting.

A daytime chart, such as the sample form included in the Appendix, should be used to record times and dates for urination and bowel movements. This chart can also be used during and after training, as needed to monitor performance and progress.

After keeping this data chart for two weeks, patterns of elimination times should become evident. At this point, begin the teaching process by routinely taking the person to the bathroom five to fifteen minutes before the times indicated on the chart. If the person needs more time to relax and focus attention to task, toileting time needs to occur several minutes before elimination usually occurs. If the elimination response is relatively quick, that time can be shorter.

Some families and teachers have difficulty fitting toileting schedules into their own routines. Having a well-defined schedule will be effective only when that agenda is followed consistently. Less structured caretakers may find a natural schedule easier to follow. A natural schedule consists of a timeframe determined by naturally occurring events such as meals, certain activities, and periods of rest or sleep.

CASE EXAMPLE

Robby's family was very active and did not adhere to a rigid schedule for meals or activities. They tried toileting him on a time schedule, but were often in the middle of an activity when it was time to toilet. This upset everyone, so Robby used the toilet upon waking, after meals, before trips in the car, and before and after active play.

CAUTION !!!

Avoid using an elaborate data collection chart when you already know the times of day your child urinates or has a bowel movement. Such charting systems are for use when you are unsure of those times or when they vary significantly from day to day.

Having scheduled toileting times serves two purposes. First, using a preplanned agenda ensures that the person will access the toilet during the times elimination is most likely to occur. This increases the probability that the program will be successful. Scheduling also builds upon the learner's strong preference for routine and adds predictability to these new behavioral expectations. When these activities are anticipated, less resistance occurs. Scheduled activities need to be effectively communicated in order to have a positive influence on training.

Communication Structures

Each person with autism has unique needs and skill levels. This must be considered when developing ways to communicate information about toileting routines. Supplement any spoken cues with visual cues to use visual strengths and concrete thinking as a foundation for understanding and cooperation. If the person effectively communicates using pictures or objects, incorporate these into the schedule and routine.

Beginning a toilet training program violates comfortable daily routines, sometimes presenting even more challenges. Using a visually-based schedule eases the anxiety that often accompanies these changes and prevents related misbehaviors from interfering with goals.

CASE EXAMPLE

Since he was five years old, his parents realized he needed to begin toilet training. David was easily upset by any changes in routine. They dreaded trying to start, knowing he would be very upset by these changes. David's teacher used a picture-based communication system at school. With the help of his teacher, David's parents made a simple schedule that outlined basic activities, including "potty" times. They also used a strip of pictures to show the sequence of tasks to complete in the bathroom. David responded favorably to these changes when pictures were used, but resisted toileting when there were no pictures to follow.

Rather than be viewed as a single event, toileting needs to be approached as a sequenced chain of behaviors that includes all of the behaviors preceding and following elimination. Use visual cues such as picture strips showing the sequence of behaviors to complete as part of the entire toileting process.

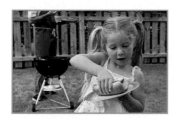 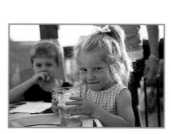 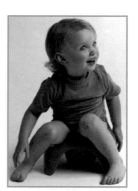 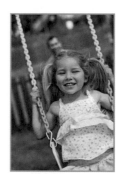

Eat   Drink   Potty   Play
                                           Outside

Approach using the toilet as an entire sequence of related behaviors for the learner to complete, including:

- Follow a visual schedule for eating foods, drinking fluids and accessing the toilet.
- Enter the bathroom and close the door when appropriate.
- Undress (only as necessary for using the toilet).
- Sit on the toilet, relax, and remain on the toilet until finished.
- Access toilet paper, wipe, and properly dispose of toilet paper.
- Get off of the toilet, flush one time, close the commode lid, and get dressed.
- Wash and dry hands, properly dispose of towel, indicate being finished with toileting, and exit the bathroom.
- Return to check what is next on the schedule and begin that activity.

Fluid Intake

Routines and schedules improve cooperation and maximize positive results from training efforts. Another tactic that significantly impacts a person's success with urinating on a regular, predictable basis is to increase and monitor the intake of fluids during training periods. Be aware of the amount of juice, water, sodas, and other fluids the person is drinking throughout the day. Also, notice when fluids are being consumed in relationship to when urination occurs. Using this knowledge, provide additional fluids about ten to fifteen minutes before scheduled toileting times. Adjust the times and amount of fluid intake so the learner is most likely to void in the commode during scheduled toilet breaks.

Undressing and Dressing

Undressing and dressing need to be included as part of the toileting routine. When planning the appropriate cues to facilitate

CAUTION !!!

- Control fluid intake in an effort to influence urination only by *increasing* the amount of fluids consumed or by changing the times fluids are made available. Avoid the temptation to *decrease* the number of times a person urinates by depriving fluids. Regular consumption of fluids, especially water, is necessary for good health.

- Avoid making someone drink an excessive amount of fluids (more than eight to ten eight-ounce glasses per day) in an effort to increase opportunities to reinforce voiding in the commode. This creates an artificial sequence of behaviors that becomes part of the person's learned routine and may also be unhealthy.

undressing, be sure to clarify removing only the clothing necessary for using the commode. Presenting unclear expectations may result in removal of all clothing when prompted to "undress." A more concise prompt may be expressed by saying "pants down" while presenting a related picture cue.

Toileting is finished after everything is restored to its original condition. This includes related dressing behaviors. As with undressing, provide clear, concrete prompts such as saying "pants up" while showing a related picture. Independent dressing and undressing can be encouraged through the use of a procedure called backward chaining. Backward chaining involves breaking a skill into smaller steps taught in a sequence, starting with the last step in the sequence being taught first.

Flushing

Flushing can either be an exciting, fun activity or a frightening experience for someone with autism. The noise and swirling

CASE EXAMPLE

When Josh finishes using the toilet, his mom helps him pull up his pants until they are one inch from his waist. Josh finishes pulling up his pants. The next time, Mom stops helping when the pants are two inches from his waist and Josh finishes. Josh is reinforced by the sense of accomplishment each time he finishes pulling up his pants by himself.

water provide excessive stimulation to the senses. For individuals who enjoy this form of sensory input, flushing serves as a logical and natural reinforcer that follows using the toilet. For others, flushing is so upsetting that it may decrease cooperation with toileting.

CAUTION !!!

- Discourage the person from flushing before toileting is completed by using picture cues to show when flushing can be done. Without clear communication indicating when one can flush, unacceptable behaviors may be used in an effort to make this happen.
- Individuals who are overwhelmed or frightened by flushing may need to be desensitized to the noise and swirling water. This can be accomplished by pairing positive reinforcers or comforting sensations with the sound or sight of flushing.
- Another approach for dealing with fears related to flushing includes changing the final sequence of the routine to: washing hands, opening the bathroom door as an escape route, then flushing and quickly exiting the room without running.

CASE EXAMPLE

Jeanna was on a toileting schedule. She seemed to understand the concept of eliminating in the toilet and successfully used the toilet at home. However, she seldom urinated in the toilet at school and frequently wet her clothes during the bus ride home. Mom asked Jeanna's teacher to schedule a parent conference to discuss possible solutions to this situation. They shared information about her fluid intake schedules and toileting routines.

Mom discovered that Jeanna's only opportunity to consume fluids during the school day was at lunch and at late afternoon snacktime. She was placed on the toilet at the end of the school day, but she was stopping at the water fountain for long periods of time during the afternoon walk to the schoolbus. They decided to include water breaks in Jeanna's school schedule approximately fifteen minutes before her toileting times. The teacher also started using a counting game to limit the amount of water Jeanna drank on the walk to the schoolbus. She took three swallows of water, then continued on to the bus. Although they had placed restrictions on Jeanna's water consumption, they actually had increased the amount of water she was drinking each day. In addition, during their meeting, Mom and Jeanna's teacher made sure they were both using the same picture cues and routines for toileting. Jeanna responded favorably to these changes. She regularly voided in the commode at school and stopped wetting her clothes during the ride home on the schoolbus. Jeanna's toilet training program was successful because her mom and teacher worked together to analyze the problems and find solutions.

CASE EXAMPLE

Tyrone panicked everytime the toilet flushed. He covered his ears and screamed. He became so anxious in anticipation of the flushing noise. It was beginning to affect his toileting behavior. Tyrone's dad added a picture for "flush" to his toileting picture cues. Tyrone then knew when flushing would occur. This decreased his anxiety significantly, but did not stop his fear of the noise. So, his dad made a tape recording of the toilet flushing. He and Tyrone listened to the recording while the volume was turned down low. He reinforced Tyrone and showed him how to control the loudness of the flushing noise on the tape recorder. Tyrone experimented with the tape and gradually learned to tolerate flushing noises at normal loudness. He more readily overcame his fear when he was able to have some control and influence over the noise.

Handwashing

Another step in the toileting routine is handwashing. Anyone learning to use the commode should be taught to wash hands following use of the toilet. To teach acceptable handwashing, clearly communicate each step involved in the process. It may be necessary for the person to first experience the entire process of handwashing to know what it feels like.

Include the following when teaching handwashing:

- Display a sequenced strip of pictures or other appropriate cues to indicate each step to be completed.
- Use precise directions such as "use one squirt of soap."
- Provide the necessary materials, including soap, water and towels within easy reach.

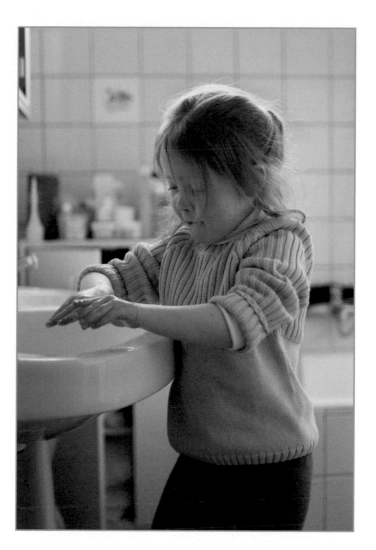

CAUTION !!!

- Avoid correcting errors by simply having the person complete the incorrect step accurately.
- Instead, correct errors by having the person repeat the last step in the sequence that was performed correctly.
- Next, complete the step that was previously done incorrectly.
- Then, continue the rest of the steps in the sequence.

CASE EXAMPLE

Jose's mom included handwashing in his toileting routine. She had a strip of pictures, covered in clear plastic, posted by the sink at Jose's eye level. These pictures were used to remind Jose to turn on the water, wet both hands, put one squirt of soap on his hands, rub his hands together, rinse, turn the water off, dry his hands and put the towel in its proper place. The first time Mom had Jose wash his hands, she showed him the steps on the picture strip and stood behind him with her hands over his, to assist him in completing the entire sequence of steps as one complete experience. This way, Jose experienced what handwashing was supposed to feel like. His mom knew that if she taught him to turn the water on as a distinct task, then do each step as if it were a separate skill to learn in isolation, Jose would need more help and assistance before he could wash his hands independently. One day Jose wet both hands but forgot to use soap. His mom showed him the picture for "wet both hands," then the picture for "use soap." She had him repeat wetting his hands, which was the last step he did correctly; then she had him put soap on his hands and continue the sequence. She knew if Jose simply corrected the error, he would not be as likely to include it in the sequence and would probably repeat the error in the future.

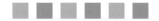

CHAPTER 4

Dressing for the Occasion

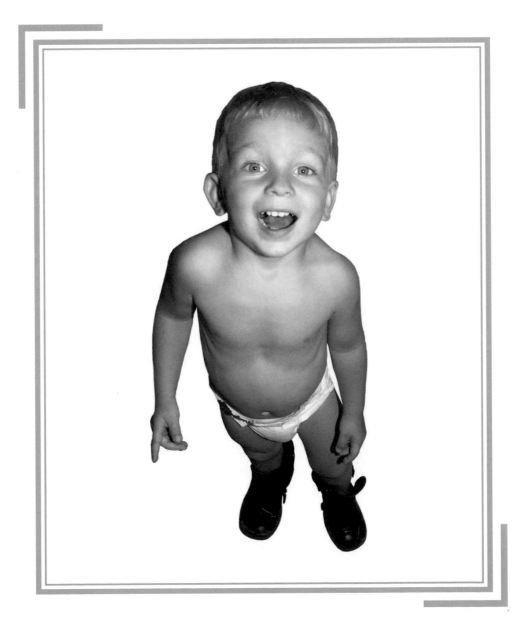

P roviding clothing and other materials that promote independence may require a few modifications to your usual selections while toilet training is in progress. These changes are usually temporary in nature. Any time choices in clothing or other materials related to toileting are being considered, a critical question to answer is "Will this help my child become more independent with toileting and self-care?" Avoid using clothing that presents a barrier to independence simply because it is attractive or it makes your caretaking easier. Teaching more independent levels of self-care usually involves a temporary increase in caretaking efforts while learning is occurring. Once a skill is established, then caretaking demands regarding that particular skill decrease significantly.

Diapers or Underpants

One significant decision that is made when toilet training begins involves the use of diapers versus underpants. This creates concern since there will continue to be times when the person eliminates in the clothing. Most underpants will not retain large amounts of wastes, resulting in time-consuming clean-up of the individual, clothing and furnishings. However, when in training, the learner must be able to feel the wetness of clothing when "accidents" occur. Diapers are designed to pull wetness away from the body and will prevent the wearer from feeling that wetness. Underpants or special training pants with extra thickness in vital areas need to be worn next to the skin. Diapers or plastic protectors may be worn outside of underpants, but should not be worn alone or against the skin.

CAUTION !!!

During training, change the learner's affected clothing anytime it is wet or soiled. Frequently feeling wet or soiled clothing against the skin for lengthy periods of time will desensitize the person to the discomfort of that sensation. This interferes with training efforts.

Outerwear

Outer clothing worn during training needs to be selected with consideration for supporting independent dressing and undressing. Avoid choosing clothing that is difficult to remove or put on, no matter how cute or attractive that outfit may be. There will be future opportunities to choose clothing based on attractiveness, once the person has improved skills and toilet training is no longer a concern.

Common clothing styles to consider choosing during training include:

- Pull-on pants or shorts with an elastic waistband
- Pants that are loosely fitted, but not too baggy
- Skirts that are loosely gathered
- Skirts or dresses that are knee-length or shorter
- Sweatpants
- Loosely fitting knit pants
- Clothing made from soft materials that are not bulky
- Shirts that are hip-length or shorter

CASE EXAMPLE

Jeffrey was always dressed in style. He wore nice-looking jeans for casual occasions and dress pants for more important events. Others frequently complimented Jeffrey's mom about how well-dressed he was. Jeffrey was learning to use the potty. Mom put training pants on him and kept his clothes changed if he had an "accident." He was responding very well to the picture schedule and seemed to understand the concept of eliminating in the toilet. He was even starting to access the toilet whenever he needed, without waiting for the scheduled times. However, Jeffrey continued to require full assistance fastening and unfastening his pants. He had a lot of problems with his jeans. Sometimes he would go into the bathroom and not be able to unfasten his pants. Unable to use the commode, he would finally just stand in the bathroom until he wet or soiled his pants. Mom began dressing him in elastic-waist jeans and pants. She realized that Jeffrey's success with independently using the toilet was more important than his stylish wardrobe. She soon discovered that he looked just as nicely dressed in easy-to-manage clothes. Watching Jeffrey become independent with toileting helped her realize she had made a wise choice that would help her son have a more successful future.

Other Items or Equipment Needed

Preparing or modifying the environment in order to promote independence and success with the complete toileting routine is critical to the effectiveness of any toilet training program. Notice every part of the environment used in the toileting routine, including the commode, sink, fixtures, toilet paper, soap, towels and other related items. Are these items within easy reach? Are measures in place to help with obtaining the right amount of toilet paper, soap or towels? Are adaptations needed to prevent harm from using hot water at the sink?

Other items, equipment, and adaptations that may be needed to promote safety and independence with toileting include:

- Plastic protectors to wear outside of underpants
- Potty seats that fit on the commode and support the child while sitting or separate potty chairs
- Stepstools that allow safe access to the sink or commode
- Soap and hand towels that can be easily managed
- Toilet paper that is convenient to obtain in appropriate amounts
- Adjustments to doors, light switches and hot water sources to promote independent, but safe use

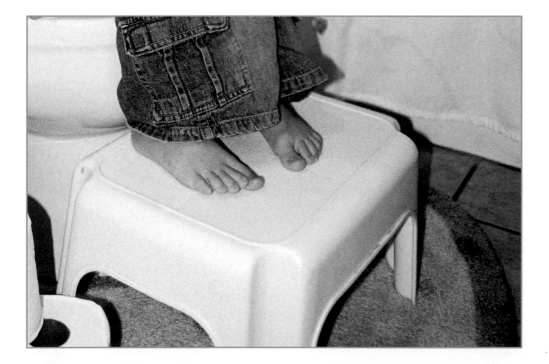

CASE EXAMPLE

Gavin used the bathroom independently. He learned this by using picture schedules. He completed the entire routine each time, including handwashing, without any help from others. When he could not remember what to do, he looked at a strip of picture cues that showed him what came next. Sometimes he turned on the hot water when washing his hands. When he tried to rinse, the water had reached such a high temperature that it burned. Dad did not want to take away any of Gavin's independence, so he addressed this concern by using picture cues and safety adjustments. First, he placed a picture showing "hot" along with the word "HOT" in big red letters next to the hot water faucet. Just in case this did not always work, he also reset the thermostat on the hot water heater from 130 degrees to 100 degrees so Gavin would not be scalded if he accidentally turned on the hot water. Gavin soon learned to only use the cold water faucet. Later, Dad changed the picture cue to a smaller one that more closely resembled the "H" on the hot water faucet. Eventually, Gavin learned to look at the letter on the faucets before turning on the water, so he no longer needed the picture cue.

Sensory Issues Related to Clothing and Other Items

While considering any necessary adaptations to equipment or other items, also analyze sensory issues related to clothing and other items connected to toilet training. Are the texture and fit of the clothing comfortable? Do the elastic and other binding parts provide support or pressure that is comfortable to that person? Some people are highly sensitive to tags, seams, or bindings in their clothing, with certain sensations being intolerable.

Is the seat on the commode or potty chair stable? Can the person get into a comfortable, secure position while seated and while washing hands? Is the texture, firmness, and fit of the seat tolerable for that individual? If the learner feels unstable or is irritated by the feel of the seat, the resultant anxiety can cause physical changes that interfere with elimination.

Does the person find the texture of the soap or towel tolerable? Being unable to tolerate the sensation from using solid or liquid soap can present a barrier to handwashing. Some people react to the scent of various soaps. If this presents a problem, experiment with different forms of soap. When making selections, remain aware of the other sensory influences such as perfumes used or the feel of different fabrics or papers. Provide soap, towels and other materials that are tolerable to that person.

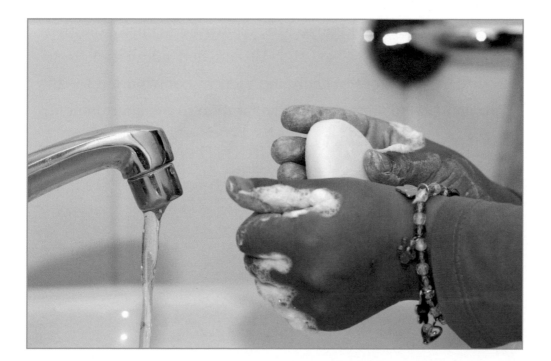

CASE EXAMPLE

Mrs. Brown was having problems potty training her daughter. Micah resisted sitting on the toilet seat. In fact, she acted as if she were terrified of sitting on the commode. She stiffened her body, screamed, and would try to hold on to Mrs. Brown anytime she was put on the commode. Of course, this would cause her to lose her balance and almost fall, which added to her fear. Mrs. Brown put a solid wooden crate at the foot of the commode. She encouraged Micah to use this crate as a stepstool for getting on the toilet. She helped Micah use the stepstool the first few times. Mrs. Brown also showed Micah how to keep her feet solidly placed on the crate while sitting on the toilet. She had carefully selected the crate's height so that it made a footrest for Micah, keeping her hips and knees flexed at a 90° angle to provide maximum support. With this in place, she felt more secure and supported while sitting on the commode. Soon Micah stopped resisting potty training. She stopped screaming and acting frightened. For a while, she continued to hold on to Mrs. Brown for security, but that eventually stopped also. Mrs. Brown had addressed these concerns by carefully analyzing factors contributing to the problem and making a simple adaptation to the environment.

Boys: Standing vs. Sitting

One final consideration when preparing the environment for toilet training boys, is the decision to teach them to stand or sit while urinating. On the surface this does not appear to be a significant issue. However, it can contribute to a variety of problems related to toileting. Carefully planning the precise behaviors to be taught, including any choices to be made, such as sitting or standing when urinating, can prevent difficult behaviors from developing accidentally.

When making the choice about teaching boys to stand or sit, consider the following:

* Does the boy distinguish between when he needs to urinate and when he needs to defecate?
* Does he observe situations and make choices appropriate to that particular situation?
* Is there a male role model present whom the boy observes and tries to imitate?
* Does he have the coordination, focus, and control needed?

If the answer to any of these questions is "yes," then learning both standing and sitting may be an option. Otherwise, focus on starting with sitting on the commode.

CASE EXAMPLE

When being toilet trained, Jacob tried to mimic Dad by standing to urinate. He was easily distracted by anything he could see, especially if it moved. His extreme distractibility contributed to some big messes in the bathroom. Jacob would start urinating while standing and when distracted he would turn toward the distractor and urinate everywhere but the toilet. A seemingly logical consequence was to require Jacob to clean up the mess, but Dad knew that Jacob would not learn to control this problem by being punished afterwards. He would simply learn to clean the bathroom after toileting. Dad also realized that Jacob was so motivated to imitate his behaviors, that sitting to urinate would upset him. Dad would either have to start modeling "sitting on the commode," or find a way to teach Jacob how to pay attention and aim for the toilet bowl. He knew that Jacob learned quickly when his strong preferences were used as strengths for teaching new skills. Dad decided to build on Jacob's visual focus and strong desire to imitate. He placed a circular piece of breakfast cereal in the toilet as part of the routine for urinating. Through modeling, he taught Jacob to aim for the floating piece of cereal. Jacob remained focused on the cereal until finished and made no more messes.

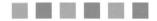

CHAPTER 5
Habit Training

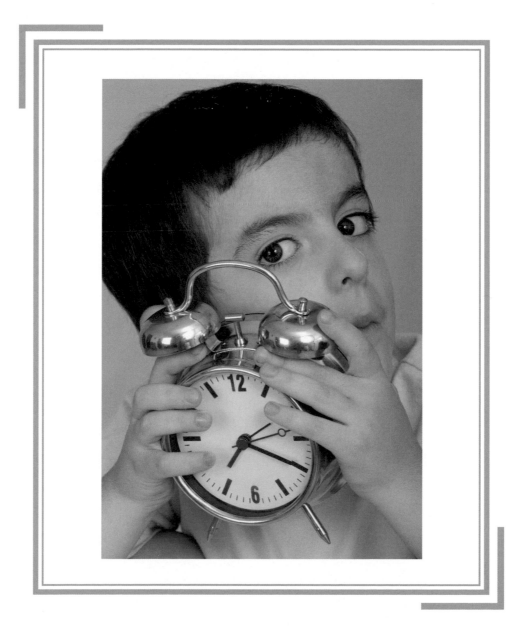

One type of toilet training available is called habit training. When providing habit training, the goal is to develop bladder and bowel control by regularly accessing toileting facilities. Eliminating in the toilet becomes a learned habit by repeating the behavior in the same way over and over. This is different from the goal of other types of toilet training. Usually the goal is teaching persons to independently access facilities when they are aware of the need to eliminate. Habit training provides a socially acceptable way to have dignity and improved personal hygiene when someone is not a good candidate for usual toilet training techniques.

When Is Habit Training Appropriate?

Habit training may be an appropriate option to consider if:

- There is no awareness of the need to urinate or defecate
- The person is older than six years of age and other training techniques have not been effective
- The individual has a mental age lower than three years
- There is no awareness or change in behavior when diapers or clothing are wet or soiled

Determining a Reasonable Schedule

The most critical part of a successful habit training program is the development and consistent use of a suitable schedule. With habit training, accurately identifying times when the learner usually urinates and has bowel movements greatly affects the program's success. Follow the procedures discussed in Chapter 3 for guidelines that support the development of sound toileting schedules.

CAUTION !!!

- When identifying times for scheduling "potty breaks," avoid selecting times that are simply more convenient. This will interfere with program success. Instead, choose times that are five to fifteen minutes before the person usually eliminates, thus creating conditions for success to be more probable.

- When using habit training, the role of regular exercise, scheduled food and drink consumption, and monitoring the types of food and drink taken become essential to success. Lack of exercise, poor eating habits, inadequate fluid intake, and physical reactions to types and quantities of food directly affect the timing of elimination. Predicting the timing of elimination is important to achieving successful results with habit training.

Developing a Routine

Developing and following a routine is an important part of habit training. Anytime the person is taken to the toilet, be sure to follow the entire toileting routine, including visual prompts, undressing, and dressing. Specific information about developing and following a toileting routine is discussed is Chapter 3.

CAUTION !!!

- Avoid asking if the person needs to use the bathroom when the schedule indicates a toileting time. Simply prompt the person that it is time to use the bathroom. Allowing the person to indicate that he or she does not need to eliminate should not be an option at this point. The cue for "potty" on the schedule is the signal that the toileting routine needs to begin.

- If the individual wets or soils clothing between scheduled toilet times, calmly help them clean up with minimal social interaction. Do not act emotional, hostile, or upset. Do not scold, lecture, or nag. Simply help the person clean up in a dignified manner and continue with the next scheduled activity. Continue to take the person to the bathroom in accordance with the schedule, following the usual routine and making no reference to the earlier "accident."

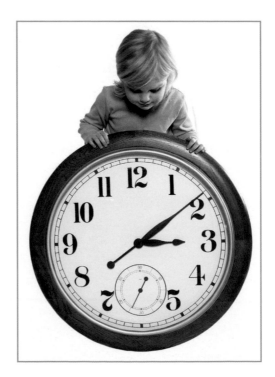

CASE EXAMPLE

Kelly's family and teacher had tried several times to toilet train her, but were unsuccessful. She did not seem to notice or feel uncomfortable when her clothes were wet or soiled. Kelly was eight years old and this was significantly affecting her socially. Other children either avoided her or treated her as if she were a baby or a novelty, especially when her diaper was wet or smelly. Kelly's teacher learned about habit training and showed the family. They could already predict the times Kelly wet or soiled her diaper, so they simply scheduled her potty breaks about ten minutes before those times. They used a picture schedule on the wall to remind themselves and Kelly when to take potty breaks. Kelly was already using a picture schedule for other activities throughout her day. Within a few weeks, Kelly was eliminating in her clothes only on rare occasions. She never did seem to learn to notice when that happened. However, she discontinued wearing diapers and the other children noticed. Kelly no longer appeared to be a baby or a novelty to them. They stopped avoiding her, since she was not so offensive anymore.

Readiness for Spontaneous Toileting

Habit training may result in preparing the individual for learning to spontaneously access the toilet. Stopping regular elimination in clothing through consistent habit training can serve to sensitize some people to the sensation of wet or soiled clothing. For some, it may serve to develop the habit of regular elimination. In this case, continence is achieved by training one's body to activate certain functions on a time schedule, rather than develop a conscious awareness of physical sensations that signal the need to eliminate. Ideally, the final goal of any form of toilet training is to develop continence, spontaneous access of toileting facilities, and independent completion of toileting routines. For some individuals, habit training can build the basic foundations for pursuing these goals. For others, it may simply add dignity, independence, and improved personal hygiene to their lives, thus removing some barriers to experiencing positive social interactions and self-sufficiency.

CASE EXAMPLE

Dustin was eleven years old and was not toilet trained. His parents had put him back in diapers after several attempts to train him. He did not even seem to notice or be uncomfortable when his clothes were wet or soiled. His parents were very frustrated and tired. As he grew older and larger, the messes in his clothing became bigger and more difficult to clean up. Dustin was included in several fifth grade classes at school. The other children noticed when he eliminated in his clothing. Some even made fun of him. Even after being cleaned up, Dustin still had an offensive odor from these accidents. His teacher and parents decided to try habit training. They identified the times Dustin usually eliminated and included those as toileting times in his picture schedule. At first, they were discouraged. Dustin was rarely eliminating in his clothes, but they did not like the idea of a future filled with taking him to the bathroom several times per day. After a few weeks, Dustin began anticipating the toileting routine and would access the bathroom unassisted when his schedule indicated. One day, a few months later, he retrieved the toilet picture from his schedule when it was not time, and used the bathroom. He had learned the concept of toileting by first developing a habit, before he learned to understand.

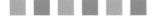

CHAPTER 6

Teaching Continence

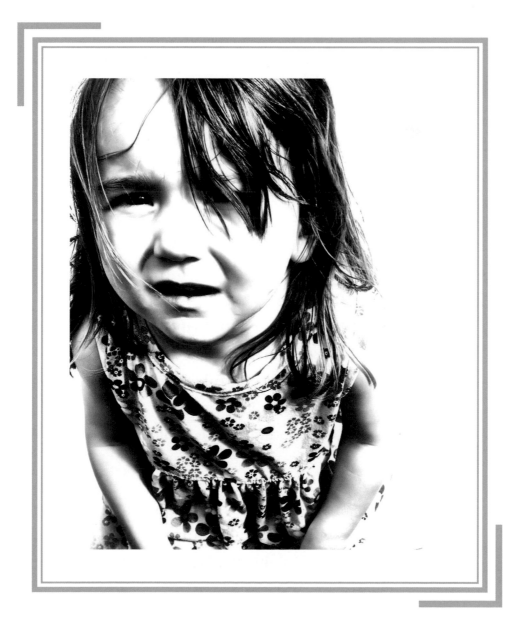

Continence is the ability to refrain from urinating or having bowel movements in one's clothing. This can be difficult to achieve for some persons with physical or mental challenges, especially for some individuals with autism. In order to truly be continent, one must develop voluntary control over bladder and bowel. Some people may have control over one but not the other. When designing a toilet training program, the question arises whether to focus on bladder control or bowel control. Although the eventual goal is to achieve both, one might ask, "Which comes first?"

Bladder Control

Usually bladder control is achieved before bowel control. Bladder control is often easier to teach since there are several opportunities for practice each day. The frequency of those learning opportunities can also be increased by providing additional fluids to drink. Bladder control can be more difficult to teach when the learner has limited awareness of the related physical sensations.

Sensations related to learning bladder control include:

- Feeling of fullness
- Feeling of voluntary control when starting urination
- Feeling of emptying the bladder
- Feeling of voluntary control over stopping urination
- Feeling of an empty bladder
- Feeling of wet clothing or bedding

Each one of the sensations related to bladder control provides cues that assist with maintaining urinary continence. Some people are incontinent due to either a lack of awareness, inattention, a decreased or absent physical feeling, or not understanding the significance or meaning related to these sensations. Habit training, as discussed in Chapter 5, can assist with meeting the toilet training needs of persons who are unaware, inattentive, or who do not understand. Habit training can also be effective with individuals who are limited by decreased or absent physical sensations. To achieve success with some learners, it may be necessary to also address other related issues.

> With some learners who have limited awareness, attention, or physical sensations, it may be necessary to teach these related behaviors as part of habit training:
>
> - How to apply physical pressure on the lower abdomen with the hands in order to empty the bladder
> - How to start urinating once seated on the toilet
> - How to count or use some other focused method after the main stream of urine has stopped to prevent impulsively leaving the toilet seat too soon

Individuals who do not have the physical control needed to empty the bladder can be taught to use their hands to apply physical pressure on the lower abdominal area over the bladder in order to facilitate emptying. People who expel small amounts of urine throughout the day may be candidates for learning this technique. This procedure would be completed whenever the person accesses the toilet as part of his or her schedule for habit training. Consult with your physician, physical therapist, or occupational therapist for further guidance or training on this technique.

Another problem that can interfere with bladder control is difficulty in beginning to urinate when positioned at the toilet. More commonly known approaches that facilitate urination include turning on the faucet to watch and listen to running water or pouring lukewarm or room temperature water on a boy's penis. The important part of any procedure used for this purpose is to decrease distractions and induce relaxation. Providing a visual and auditory focus helps eliminate the negative effects of distractions. The running water works by providing a focus while imitating a sound related to urinating.

People who do not benefit from more common methods may need greater assistance with relaxation and reducing distractions. Individuals who are highly anxious may have difficulty relaxing enough to urinate. In these situations, providing the person with comfortable, relaxing activities while on the toilet can facilitate elimination. These activities may vary greatly from person to

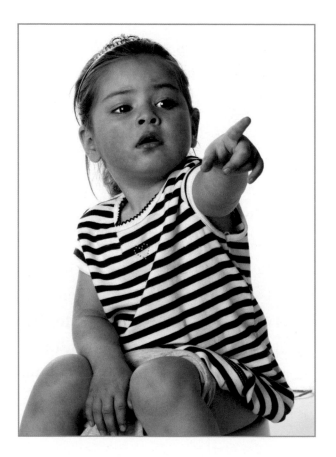

person. The solution may be to play music or look at a book or magazine. Some people may require more involved approaches such as providing a table top and a few toys. Providing a small table top is especially helpful to prevent accidentally dropping objects into the commode. It may also serve to help the person feel more secure while sitting on the toilet.

Some individuals who are inattentive or very impulsive may leave the toilet when the main part of elimination has stopped and leave before completely finishing. This behavior can result in small amounts of urine or feces getting on clothing, hands, or surface areas in the bathroom. Persons who engage in such behavior frequently have an offensive odor resulting from this action. For both social and sanitary reasons, these individuals need to be taught to delay leaving the toilet for a specific period of time after they perceive they are finished. For those who are younger or more seriously challenged, requiring them to count to ten or twenty very slowly can delay leaving the commode. If they are unable to count, have them touch each picture on their sequence of picture cues for their toileting routine before leaving the toilet, in order to create a significant delay. Others may simply look at their watch, stopwatch, timer, or a clock until ten to thirty seconds have passed.

Bowel Control

Bowel control is usually learned following bladder control. However, some individuals develop bowel control first. When developing a toileting schedule, be sure to also target the times that bowel movements occur, in order to begin teaching this important behavior. Due to the physical features that distinguish it from bladder control and the unique sensations involved, some challenging problems related to bowel control can arise, especially when training a person who has autism. Some individuals are frightened or perplexed about bodily functions they do not

CASE EXAMPLE

Ben was on a habit training schedule. He cooperated with sitting on the commode momentarily, but would impulsively jump up and look at other things in the bathroom after a few seconds. His parents had been very careful in setting up and following a schedule that reflected the times he usually eliminated. Sometimes the schedule was so accurate that Ben would urinate on the floor or himself as he was moving away from the toilet or wandering around the bathroom. Once he jumped up it was extremely difficult to get him to sit down on the toilet again. Ben's parents decided to place a small plastic table in front of him as soon as he sat on the toilet. They positioned the table so the top was over his lap and he could play with items placed on the table. They also played classical music softly in the background, dimmed the bathroom lights to add to the relaxing mood, and put some of Ben's toys on the table. They selected toys that interested Ben but did not excite him. These toys could be accessed only at bathroom time. These strategies helped Ben stay in postion and focus his attention long enough to complete elimination. When they heard him urinate in the toilet, they counted aloud to ten very slowly, then removed the table, prompted Ben to get up, flush, dress, and wash his hands.

understand. One boy with autism stated that he recalled trying to keep from having a bowel movement "because I thought my insides were coming out." Another young man said the pressure and weight of a diaper that was filled with waste felt calming to him and having a bowel movement in the toilet felt very upsetting because that feeling was almost the opposite experience of the calming feeling.

CAUTION !!!

When selecting cues and picture symbols to present, be extremely aware of the literal, concrete interpretation that many people with autism exhibit. For individuals who are very concrete thinkers, choose a picture that clearly symbolizes exactly what needs to happen.

When exploring solutions to challenging behaviors regarding bowel control:

- Identify the need that is being met by the person's current performance or behavior.
- Explore acceptable ways to meet those needs while gradually moving closer to the desired behavior.
- Carefully select picture cues to clarify expectations.
- Use stories describing people engaging in the correct behavior to teach that behavior, being careful to provide precise, concrete descriptions (discussed in Chapter 11).

CASE EXAMPLE

Gary responded to picture cues exactly as they were presented. When being toilet trained, he would get off the toilet and, when relaxed, have a bowel movement in the living room. He then took the waste and put it in the toilet. That's where the pictures cued him to put it! His parents arranged for a more relaxing potty break and changed the picture that showed waste in the toilet to a cue showing waste being expelled while sitting on the commode. Gary followed the new cues and was successful.

CASE EXAMPLE

Chris was almost nine years old, but he never seemed uncomfortable in a soiled diaper. He actually seemed to enjoy it. He quickly learned bladder control, but was having no success with bowel control. Mom resorted to putting him back in a diaper because of the mess he made when he soiled his underpants. Chris enjoyed any type of touch or activity that provided a feeling of deep, firm pressure being applied to him. She realized that Chris probably liked the pressure and weight from his soiled diaper, but had to get him toilet trained. She made a toileting schedule that targeted the times he had bowel movements. She made a picture schedule to help with the routine and provided relaxing activities during toileting. Most importantly, Mom helped Chris gradually adjust to the feeling of defecating in the toilet by first cutting a long slit in the middle of his diaper so the waste would fall into the commode, but he would still feel the snugness of his diaper. Over the next few weeks, she gradually cut away more of the diaper until it no longer provided the snug feeling that had interfered with his being successful with toilet training. She made sure that he also had scheduled times to receive deep pressure sensations periodically throughout the day and on request.

CASE EXAMPLE

Allen was seven years old and had bladder control. He continued to resist having bowel movements, either in the toilet or in his clothes. Sometimes he held himself for two to four days, becoming very anxious and physically resistant if he sensed the urge to defecate. When he could no longer resist, he would become very upset and even nauseous afterward. Allen's parents thought he did not understand this was a normal bodily function and was frightened by the feelings he was experiencing. Physical resistance only served to make the experience more uncomfortable and frightening. Allen was very responsive to pictures and books, so they went to the library and found a book with pictures that showed and explained how the digestive system functions. They also wrote a specific story for Allen that described a boy responding appropriately to these experiences. Allen's parents read this story to him every day. They also provided books, magazines, and music when Allen was in the bathroom. They made sure he ate enough fiber, drank adequate amounts of water, and engaged in activities that provided regular physical exercise. Allen stopped resisting and began having bowel movements in the commode. He did not seem frightened or anxious about this anymore.

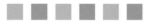

CHAPTER 7

Communicating the Need to Use the Toilet

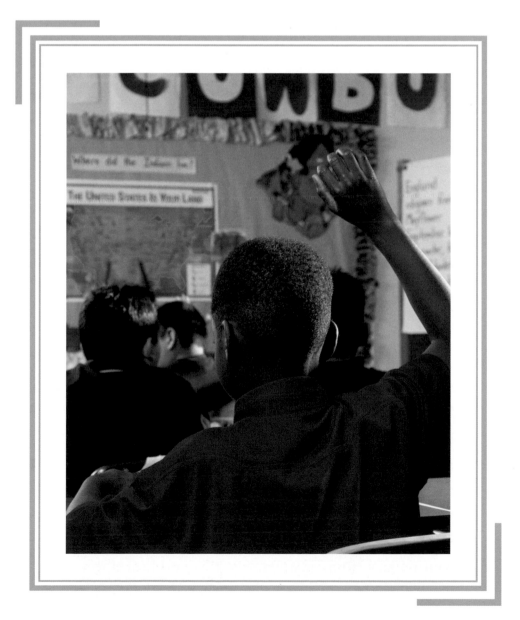

Many individuals with autism have limitations that impact their ability to communicate with others. Effective communication is essential when teaching toileting routines. Additionally, individuals who rely on someone else to assist with completing those routines must be able to let their caretaker know when help is needed.

Some difficulties experienced by people with autism that may impact communication needed for toilet training include:

- Difficulty filtering out extraneous information
- Disorganization
- Easily distracted
- Difficulty attaching meaning to what is heard
- Problems focusing attention
- Literal or concrete interpretations of language
- Limited understanding or use of language

Alternate Forms of Communication

When individuals' experience communication that is limited, identify and use alternate ways for them to focus attention, understand, respond to, and spontaneously initiate interactions with others. Alternative forms of communication furnish methods for communicating that are acceptable and effective. Alternative communication systems that build upon the user's skills and strengths provide powerful approaches that increase understanding and expression. When planning toilet training for someone who has limited communication skills, include alternative communication systems that utilize common characteristics such as preference for routine and ritual, visual strengths, and literal thinking.

Some alternative forms of communication that use visual strengths, preference for routine and ritual, and literal thinking include:

- Object swap
- Picture exchange, using photographs, pictures, or picture symbols with words
- Printed words

Refer to the Appendix for resources that teach how to develop and implement the alternative communication systems that are appropriate for various individuals. Select the approach that matches the needs and strengths of the person being toilet trained. Use the system consistently throughout the training process.

Availability of Communication

An effective communication system must continue to be available to the learner following completion of toilet training. All of us need to be able to interact with others to identify the location of restroom facilities when in unfamiliar settings. Children or others who are dependent on caretakers should be able to adequately indicate the need to access the restroom in any situation. In order to do this, alternative forms of communication must continue to be available at all times.

CAUTION !!!

Failure to provide alternative forms of communication may significantly interfere with toilet training. Be sure the system that is used is appropriately matched to the individual's needs and abilities.

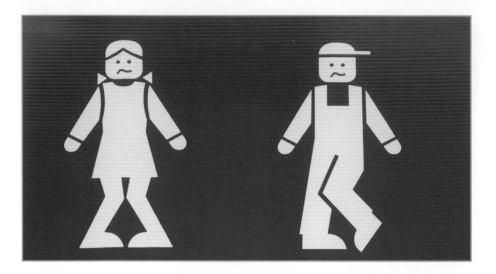

CASE EXAMPLE

Devon's parents had successfully toilet trained him. They started his training by using a picture schedule and a toileting routine. Devon responded favorably to the pictures on his schedule and the picture sequences used to remind him to complete each step of the routine. Eventually, he was accessing the bathroom independently and no longer needed his picture symbols as part of this routine. However, he occasionally wet or soiled his clothes when in the community or unfamiliar situations. This upset Devon and perplexed his parents. They decided to provide him with a pocket-size wallet that contained a few basic picture symbols to assist him with communicating when he could benefit from these extra supports. Devon began using the pictures to communicate the need to use the restroom when they were on community outings or in unfamiliar situations. He stopped having "accidents" when he had the pictures to use. Although Devon was able to verbalize, talking did not meet all of his communication needs when he was in situations that created high levels of excitement or anxiety. Some of that anxiety was decreased with the reassurance that he could request a restroom break whenever needed.

How to Respond to Communication Efforts

When teaching toileting skills, the vital role of communication is often overlooked or underestimated by caretakers who are so familiar with the learner that they do not recognize many nonverbal behaviors as efforts to communicate. People who do not consistently speak to provide information to others may rely on behaviors such as gestures, pointing, pulling, pushing, grabbing, or similar strategies that do not include spoken words. This nonverbal communication may also include vocalizations such as whining, fussing, crying, whimpering, screaming, or other noises that do not include attempts to speak words. When such behaviors are used for communication purposes, they should be followed by a response from the receiver. The person who is attempting to communicate needs to understand that relaying information is a very powerful process that results in responses.

CAUTION !!!

Avoid ignoring any efforts by an individual to communicate, even when these attempts are not ideal. Failure to respond to such overtures may result in the person resorting to unacceptable behavior or avoiding future communication attempts.

When a gesture or other behavior that is not part of a person's alternative communication system is used in an attempt to communicate the need to access the toilet, respond by pairing the preferred form of communication with helping the person obtain what was being requested. Pairing the acceptable form of communication, such as a picture, with obtaining desired goals will promote understanding and use of the preferred system.

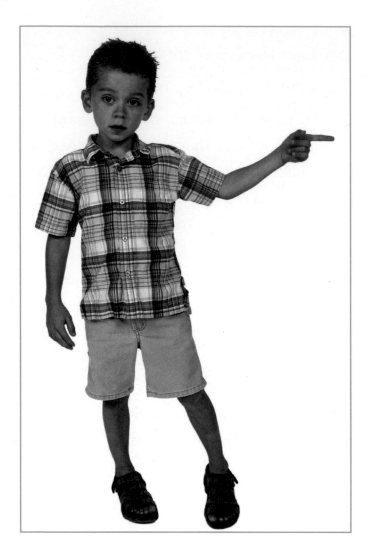

Demanding Communication can be a Step Backwards

The ultimate goal of toilet training is for an individual to sponta-neously access the toilet and complete the routine independently, without assistance from others. Once an individual has achieved this goal, demanding communication before beginning the routine can be a step backwards. Allow the person to spontaneously access the toilet without first having to ask permission. However,

CASE EXAMPLE

Maurice was being potty trained by his teacher. He did not like having wet or soiled diapers and seemed to understand the concept of using the toilet. Sometimes, Maurice would leave an ongoing activity and go stand within three feet of the door. Others did not always know what he wanted and he would wet or soil his pants. His teacher began giving him the "potty" picture when he stood by the door and would then take him to the restroom. She began consistently using the picture for scheduled potty breaks also. After several days, Maurice began retrieving the "potty" picture before standing by the door. Everyone knew what he was telling them and he stopped having "accidents" in his clothes.

for some caretakers, avoiding the uncertainty created when someone suddenly bolts out the door to go to the restroom is a significant priority. Under these circumstances, set up a routine whereby the person places a picture or printed word in a pre-defined location by the door to inform authority figures of the intended destination when leaving the room.

CAUTION !!!

Avoid setting up routines whereby an individual draws excessive attention from peers or others when leaving to access the restroom or engaging in other necessary departures. When planning such routines, select strategies that are subtle, yet communicate the necessary information in a clear manner.

CASE EXAMPLE

Brandon was fully included in a third-grade class at school. He had recently been toilet trained. During class he would sometimes jump up and bolt for the door when he needed to access the toilet. His teacher told Brandon that it was not acceptable for him to do this without asking permission. Brandon was doing well to recognize the sensations that signaled the need to use the restroom and respond accordingly. He did not have much time to react once he recognized the signals to use the restroom. When he began trying to comply with his teacher's expectation to request permission, he frequently wet or soiled his clothing before making it to the restroom. He began bolting for the door as he frantically yelled, "Gotta pee!" without waiting for a response. His teacher decided to try a different approach that would inform her of his destination while allowing him the time he needed to reach the restroom. She provided each student with a namecard and placed a pocket that read "Restroom" next to the door. When anyone in her class needed to access the restroom, the student placed his namecard in the pocket and left the room without disturbing the class. Brandon's namecard was on his desktop as a reminder. He consistently used the card and stopped disrupting the class and having "accidents."

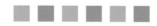

CHAPTER 8

When Toilet Training Is Successful

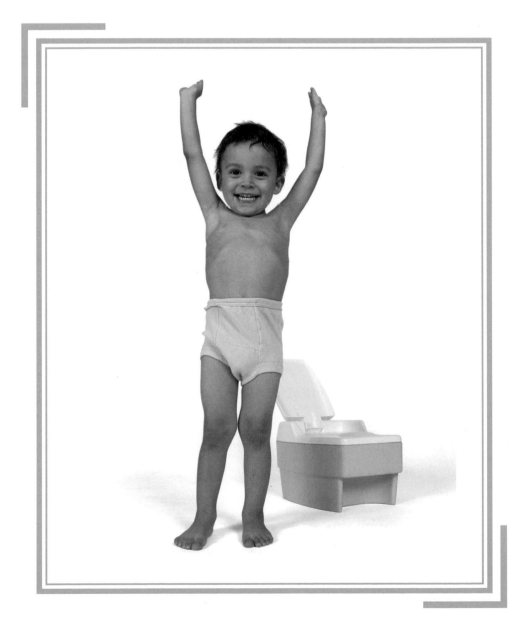

Toilet training programs are used to teach individuals to eliminate in the toilet. The final goal of this training is for the learner to access the toilet as needed without assistance from other people. For some persons who are dependent on caretakers to assist with daily living skills, the goal is to spontaneously communicate the need to access the toilet, thus minimizing the time spent on toileting throughout each day.

Toilet training is not complete until the person learns to:

- Indicate the need to access the toilet without relying on cues or reminders from other people
- Access the toilet independently when needed, without relying on cues or reminders from other people
- Complete the toileting routine independently
- Rely on visual cues, instead of verbal prompts, when reminders are needed

---

Throughout the training experience there will be successes. Rewarding those successes with positive reinforcement is a critical part of the training process. However, it is very important to plan any reward or reinforcement in advance, so it can be used effectively. Many individuals with autism react negatively with surprise, fear, confusion, or dislike when presented with reinforcement that is emotional or not logically related to the behavior it follows. Try to maintain a calm, non-emotional approach throughout the training process. Keep reinforcement low key and as a natural part of the toileting process. Being able to flush is often the most natural reinforcer for many persons who successfully eliminate in the commode. Genuine praise that is not overly emotional or loud can also be rewarding.

When and How to Reinforce

Any reinforcement needs to be provided after the entire toileting routine is completed. Providing reinforcement following completion of each part of the routine may serve to interrupt completion of the entire sequence.

> ### CAUTION !!!
>
> Avoid loud, emotional displays when reinforcing acceptable behavior. This may frighten or otherwise upset someone who is highly sensitive and may interfere with training.

Some people need more than natural reinforcement such as flushing or praise to be motivated to complete the entire toileting routine. Under these circumstances, add one final picture at the end of the toileting picture sequence that shows the reward the person will receive when finished.

Including a picture of the reward at the end of the picture sequence clearly communicates:

- The reward to work for
- How to obtain the reward
- What steps need to be completed before obtaining that reward
- When the reward will be available

CAUTION !!!

Avoid relying on spoken words to present potential rewards. This can lead to misunderstanding, confusion, and unacceptable behaviors. Use visual strategies for presenting information about potential rewards.

The Importance of Environmental Structure

Throughout the toilet training process, careful structuring of the environment promotes increased progress and reduces frustration for everyone involved. However, when training is complete, the environmental structure remains important for success to continue at a more independent level. Removing the structure and support provided by visual cues should not be a goal of training. These serve as foundations for success for visual thinkers and should remain in place. Changing the appearance of those visual cues may be appropriate, but avoid abruptly ending the use of visual prompts. The visual structures can be refined to be less obvious and more natural looking as the learner develops independence.

CASE EXAMPLE

After successfully toilet training Sue, Mom removed all of the pictures she used for training. Mom soon realized that Sue was skipping steps such as flushing and handwashing. Sometimes she left the water running. Scolding and reminding her did not help. Mom had to stay with Sue and remind her to complete each step. She posted the pictures in the bathroom again, and Sue started completing all of the routine independently. Later, Mom posted a smaller version of those pictures.

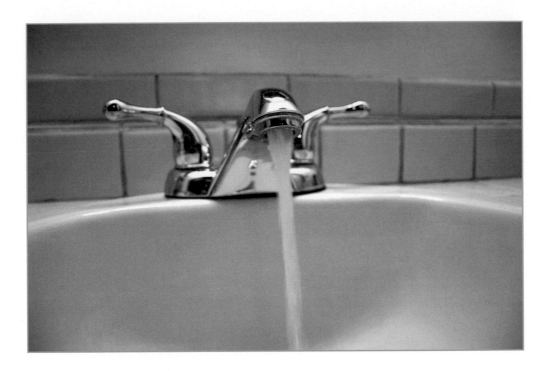

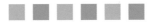

CHAPTER 9

Toileting in Unfamiliar Environments

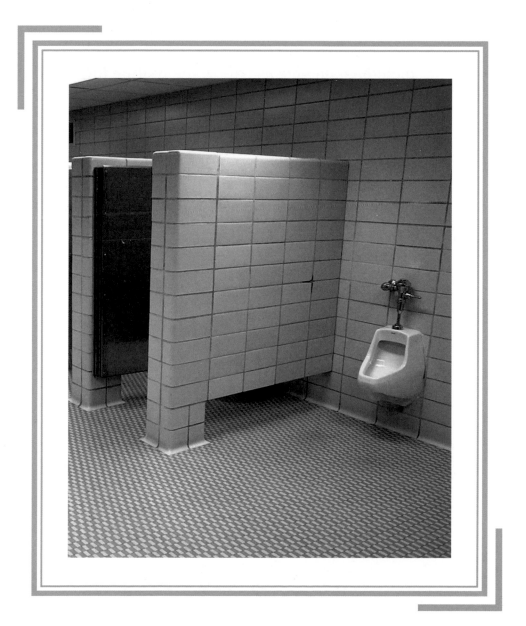

R egular routines that are easily accomplished can become difficult challenges in unfamiliar settings or under unusual conditions. A person may be able to consistently complete toileting routines independently at home and at school, but may wet and soil clothing when out in the community. Preparing in advance for the possible need to access restrooms when in the community, in unfamiliar settings, or under unusual circumstances, will help prevent significant problems.

During uncommon or exciting situations, prepare for meeting toileting needs with minimal problems by:

- Including toileting as part of the routine for departure before leaving home or school
- Making yourself aware of the location of restroom facilities upon arrival
- Carrying easily accessible picture cues or other communication supports that are part of the toileting routine

Locating Restrooms in New Environments

Upon arrival at an unfamiliar destination, look for signs that indicate the locations of public restroom facilities. If unable to find any posted signs or maps, quietly inquire about the location of those facilities. Knowing in advance where to access accommodations will help any necessary trips to the restroom happen more smoothly, without upsetting disturbances or frustrating delays. This will also prevent the individual from developing excessive anxiety over the use of public restrooms.

CAUTION !!!

- Avoid postponing locating the restroom facilities, in hopes the individual will not require their use. This will only serve to make any toileting experiences in the community more stressful and hurried, resulting in higher levels of anxiety that can interfere with self-control and cooperation.

- Avoid loud, emotional, or novel requests for locating restroom facilities. Unusual interactions can direct the individual's focus toward accessing the restroom immediately, rather than when truly needed. Subtly ask for this information without making an issue of it.

Communicating the Need to Toilet

Regardless of whether a person is comfortable with speaking verbally or using an alternative communication system, expressing the need to go to the bathroom can be a difficult challenge when surroundings are unfamiliar or exciting. Under such circumstances, carrying a few pictures related to the outing's activities and personal needs can help the person understand and express wants, needs, thoughts, or ideas.

CAUTION !!!

- If someone is unable to adequately communicate in a particular situation, unacceptable behaviors in the form of noncompliance, disruptiveness, panic attacks, tantrums, or aggression may occur. This is particularly evident when persons who have experienced the satisfaction of effective communication in some previous settings are not provided with the supports needed for adequate communication across all situations.

- Recognize that someone who is verbal and experiences significant levels of anxiety may have difficulty speaking when exposed to unfamiliar, exciting, or unusual situations or conditions. Under these circumstances, avoid demanding or expecting verbalizations. Instead, carry some basic back-up supports, such as a few pictures, to aid with communication.

Adjusting Toileting Routines to New Situations

Toileting routines in public restrooms or unfamiliar facilities may differ from the routines used at home or school. Sometimes these differences seem minor, such as rougher toilet paper or taller commodes. At other times the differences, such as too many people, an entire row of urinals that periodically flush automatically or noisy blow dryers with no "off" switch, can be overwhelming. When overwhelmed or surprised by such differences some people panic, tantrum, or react with other unacceptable behaviors.

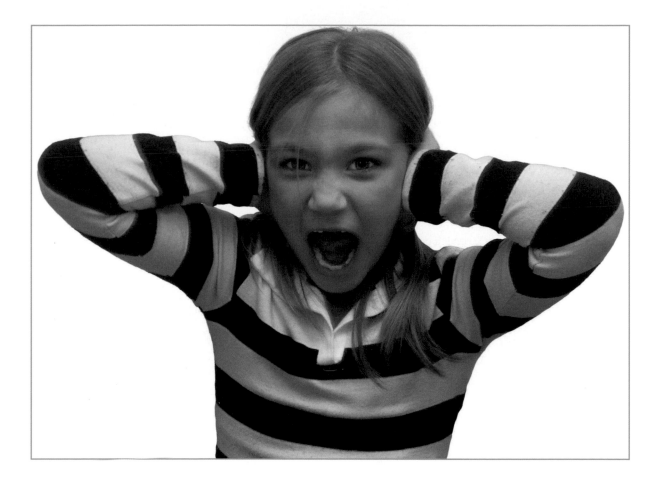

To avoid unpleasant reactions to differences in routines:

- Anticipate surprises or areas of difficulty for that individual and carry a few pictures to aid with understanding the differences.
- Carry familiar items, such as a small hand towel or soft toilet paper, in situations where differences are not tolerated.
- Turn surprises into a game by changing uncertainties into anticipated and predicted unknowns.
- Explore and practice responses to differences in advance.

Survival Kits for Community Outings

With planning and preparation, venturing into the community or unfamiliar places can be a rewarding and educational experience. As with any adventure, packing and carrying a survival kit increases the probability that the experience will be positive.

Survival kits for use during outings with someone who has autism should contain various items or materials needed to:

- Promote communication during anxiety-ridden, upsetting, or otherwise difficult situations
- Provide personal data and identification that may be needed in an emergency, including information to prevent misunderstanding regarding limitations in behaviors or communication that may appear to others as offensive or threatening
- Basic items needed for personal hygiene, if the usual public offerings are intolerable to the individual
- A few basic items that provide comfort to the person, such as a favorite toy, small blanket, wristband, snack items, walkman with headphones, book, earplugs, or other readily portable objects that are calming

---

CASE EXAMPLE

Mary was ten years old. She did not like loud noises. She would panic, scream, and become physically combative when the only way to dry her hands was with loud, uncontrollable blow dryers. When Mary became upset, Mom scolded her and took her by the arm to make her comply. This only disturbed Mary more and made her misbehavior worse. Mom dreaded taking her to the restroom. She decided to prepare a survival kit including foam earplugs that Mary had practiced wearing at home, pictures to cue her to complete her toileting routine, disposable wet towlettes, and personal identification noting that she has autism, which can result in difficulty understanding, talking, and remaining calm at times. Mary kept her survival kit in a fanny pack worn on the front of her waist. This helped her remember to use the items in it. The next time they were out, Mom noticed the blow dryer while entering the restroom. She stopped, showed Mary the blow dryer and used pictures for her to choose between wearing the earplugs or using the towlettes to wash her hands. Mary chose to use both items. Then Mom showed her the toilet picture and she completed her toileting routine with no further problems. Instead of washing her hands, Mary used the moist towlettes while standing far away from the hand dryer.

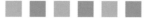

CHAPTER 10

Teaching Nighttime Continence

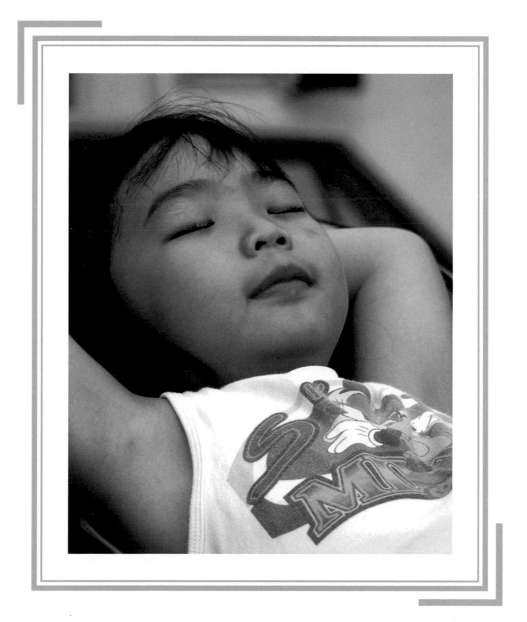

The ability to maintain bladder and bowel control at night requires a different set of skills from those needed when one is awake. Nighttime toilet training can be considered once the person achieves a reasonable amount of success with daytime toileting routines.

When to Begin Nighttime Training

Individuals who independently complete toileting routines during waking hours but wet the bed at night are good candidates for nighttime training. Those having bladder and bowel control for most of the day with occasional wetting or soiling accidents, or those who just need occasional reminders to flush, wash hands, or turn the water off, are also ready for learning control during the night. For someone who is habit trained, nighttime training may be appropriate if scheduled toileting is successful in preventing soiling or wetting clothes most of the time.

CAUTION !!!

- Avoid trying to toilet train someone at night when frequent or regular wetting or soiling of clothes in the daytime is still a problem.
- Avoid trying to teach nighttime and daytime bladder and bowel control all at once. Address daytime needs first.

How to Teach Nighttime Continence

To remain continent through the night, one must either prevent elimination from occurring or learn how to respond in a timely manner to sensations that signal the need to access the toilet. The most effective approaches to nighttime toilet training incorporate both of these strategies.

When teaching nighttime continence the learner should:

- Limit fluid intake in the evenings and rely on daytime consumption to provide adequate fluids.
- Consume no fluids for two to three hours before bedtime.
- Have a regular time for going to bed each night, including weekends and holidays.
- Have a consistent bedtime routine.
- Toilet immediately before going to bed.
- Toilet anytime awakened during the night.
- Toilet immediately upon waking in the morning.

Potty Breaks During the Night

Some individuals sleep so soundly they are not roused by the urge to eliminate. This only presents a problem when restricting intake of food and drink does not prevent nighttime elimination. For these individuals, nighttime toilet training may need to include a care provider waking them in the night and taking them to the toilet. Usually one potty break during the night is enough to control this problem. However, it may be necessary to try several different times for toileting before an ideal time is identified.

Special Aids

Specific aids are available that will rouse persons who need assistance with nighttime training. These mechanical devices set off a loud alert or warning sound once the person begins urinating and the device detects small amounts of wetness. The apparatus is intended to startle the person into an awakened state and interrupt elimination until he can get out of bed and go to the

CASE EXAMPLE

Lance was toilet trained in the daytime but still wet the bed most nights. Mom made sure he stopped drinking and eating three hours before bedtime. Lance used the toilet immediately before going to bed. When Mom checked him at 11:00 p.m. as she was retiring for the night, he was dry. She decided to start taking him to the toilet in the middle of the night and set her alarm for 2:00 a.m. This was difficult after working all day; besides, Lance had already wet the bed. Then Mom decided to take him to the potty at 11:00 p.m., just before she went to bed. He used the toilet and was dry the next morning. Mom did not even have to rouse him fully awake. Lance stopped wetting the bed and Mom was sleeping through the night.

toilet. The eventual goal of using such tools is to teach the person to waken when the urge to eliminate is sensed. If the alarm is upsetting or contributes to confusion or disorientation, these types of devices may not be as effective with persons who have autism. Being awakened in such an exciting manner may interfere with returning to a sound sleep. If these are not issues that impact the individual being trained, then such devices may be a viable option to explore. However, it may be less stressful with fewer resultant problems, such as inability to return to sleep, if the person were simply habit trained at night by being roused to toilet at a scheduled time that complements the care provider's normal routine.

CAUTION !!!

Avoid using approaches that result in increased anxiety or fear reactions. Instead, identify the strategies that were effective during daytime training and incorporate them as part of the nighttime routine.

CHAPTER 11
Support Strategies

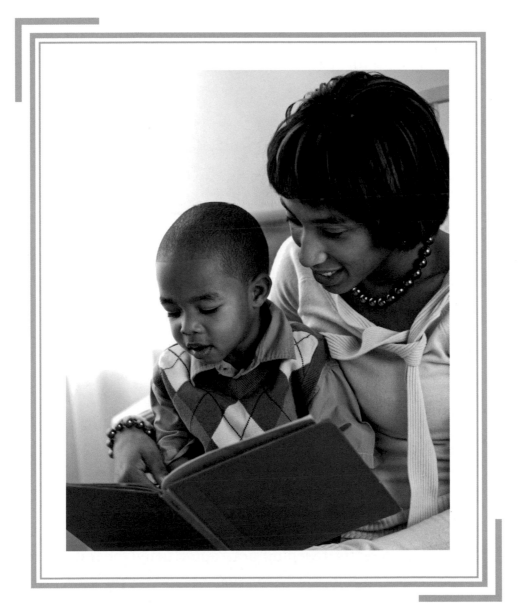

The support strategies explored in this chapter are applications of novel techniques that are often effective with individuals who have autism. These strategies are meant to supplement the approaches discussed throughout this book to hasten progress and increase understanding of expectations and routines involved with toilet training.

Modeling

Modeling involves the learner watching someone else complete a behavior correctly, in hopes the learner will accurately imitate that same behavior. For persons with autism to learn the correct steps of a behavior through modeling, their attention must be directed to the important parts of the behavior they are observing.

CAUTION !!!

When the learner's attention is not directed, the focus may be averted to novel details, overlooking and failing to imitate relevant parts. Always point out the important points to notice when using modeling as a teaching strategy.

Stories That Teach

Another highly effective, novel approach for teaching skills is to develop stories that descibe someone engaging in the desired behavior. These teaching stories should be written in the present tense and describe the relevant steps in the skill as they are being carried out. Make each story into a small book. Illustrating teaching stories with pictures can also be a powerful support for some people. Read the teaching story about using the toilet to the person each day. Allow the individual to access the book anytime he chooses. For those who cannot read, supplement the most relevant printed words in the story with the pictures that are used as cues during the toileting routine. Present only one step, using one to three sentences, per page. Describe steps in a positive way without lecturing, nagging, or describing what to avoid doing. A sample story about toileting is included in the Appendix.

Pre-teaching

Pre-teaching is another novel approach for teaching skills in a more effective manner. Pre-teaching consists of providing clear reminders to the learner immediately before the skill is to be used. The reminders may be verbal, visual, or physical; however, to be most effective, provide visual reminders that build on the individual's preferences and strengths.

Preteaching can be provided most effectively by:

- Presenting a picture cue to remind the learner about the next task or any changes to anticipate
- Presenting a sequenced strip of picture cues to remind the learner about the steps for completing the task
- Reading a teaching story about the task or routine to be completed immediately prior to starting that task
- Watching a videotape of the task being completed correctly

CAUTION !!!

Be extremely careful to avoid videotaping parts of the toileting routine or any other self-help routines showing people undressed. Legal liability could result from showing partial nudity or acts perceived as lewd.

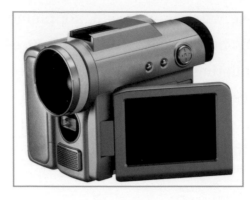

CASE EXAMPLE

Nathan was frequently resistant to efforts toward toilet training. At times he cooperated, but other days he tried to grab everything he saw, ignoring the toileting routine. Occasionally he became combative when Mom tried to physically redirect him to toileting tasks. If he looked at the commode when he went into the bathroom, he flushed the toilet. If he looked at the sink, he turned on the faucet and played in the water. If he saw the bathtub first, he started taking off his clothes and tried to climb into the tub. Efforts to interfere resulted in screaming, pulling away, aggression, and tantrums. Mom decided to write a story about Nathan following his toileting routine. She worded the story as if he did each step of the tasks correctly. Before Nathan walked into the bathroom to begin his toileting routine, she read the story to him, pointing out pictures that matched the ones she used in his strip of visual cues. Then she handed him a picture of the toilet and continued to direct his attention to the picture as he entered the bathroom. As each task in the routine was ending, she handed him the picture to cue him to start the next task. When Mom carefully directed his attention by using pictures and the story for pre-teaching, Nathan completed his routine with no problems.

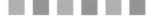

CHAPTER 12

Common Problems and Solutions Associated with Toilet Training Persons with Autism

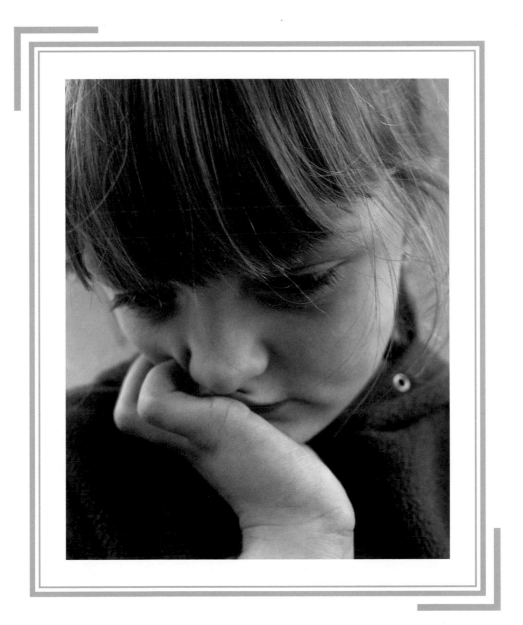

The issues explored in this chapter involve special problems experienced when toilet training persons with autism. The strategies proposed are brief guidelines using techniques explored in this book. The case examples describe solutions that worked in specific situations.

Fear of the Bathroom

Some individuals have difficulty with toilet training due to being afraid to enter the bathroom. This seems to happen more frequently in school and public restrooms, possibly due to the size, coldness, noise factors, increased numbers of people, and unfamiliarity.

Fear of the bathroom may be addressed by:

- Desensitizing the person to the bathroom by pairing it with pleasant, calming, or positive experiences
- Using picture cues to direct the person's focus
- Using positive reinforcement for accessing the bathroom

Fear of Sitting on the Toilet

Some individuals, especially children, react negatively to sitting on the commode. Reactions may range from whimpering, fussing, or showing increased agitation, to physically resisting touching the toilet. Negative reactions may be in response to finding the

CASE EXAMPLE

Chris was afraid of the bathroom at school. His teacher, Ms. Long, used a habit training schedule. His picture schedule was posted in the classroom. When it was time for Chris to potty, he walked with Ms. Long down the hall to the restroom. As soon as he entered the restroom, he began running around the room, yelling, hitting the walls, flushing the urinals, and hitting Ms. Long if she was in his way. This escalated to Ms. Long physically trying to make him enter the stall. Usually Chris resisted, becoming more assaultive. Most of the time, he would become so noncompliant and aggressive that Ms. Long would physically restrain him on the bathroom floor until he was calm. The restraints lasted from fifteen minutes to two hours. Of course, with his toileting schedule, this happened several times each day. Some days Ms. Long felt as if all she did was spend the day restraining Chris in the bathroom. Both of them were frustrated, emotionally spent, and exhausted. A behavior consultant suggested taking pictures to the restroom for communicating "sit on toilet," "wash hands," and "go to class." Chris responded well to the pictures. He used the restroom correctly with no problems and was not restrained anymore.

feel of the porcelain intolerable, feeling unstable while on the toilet, being afraid of the noise or the swirling water, or being afraid of falling into or touching the water.

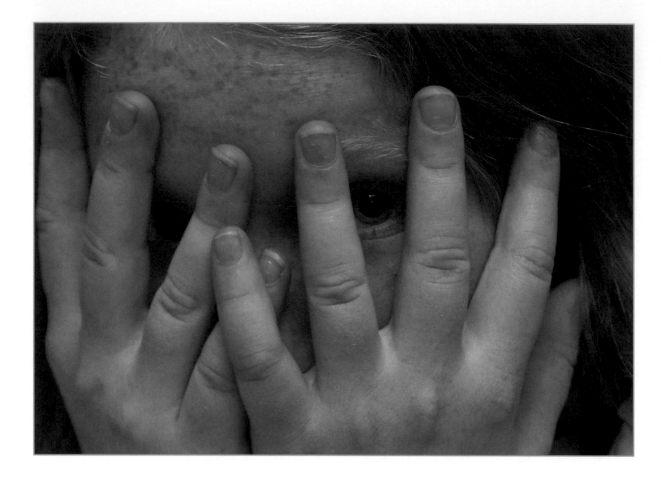

Fear of sitting on the toilet may be addressed by:

- Providing foot rests or other stabilizing devices such as potty seats that allow the person to sit securely with his feet resting flat on a solid surface
- Providing a small table that fits over the person's lap while sitting, to provide stabilizing support and direct attention to preferred tasks while on the toilct
- Desensitizing the person to the toilet by pairing it with pleasant, calming, or positive experiences such as music
- Using a separate potty chair
- Providing positive reinforcement for accessing the toilet

CASE EXAMPLE

Cameron screamed and physically resisted when Mom attempted to put him on the toilet. Using a potty seat did not alter his reaction and he refused to sit on a separate potty chair. Mom decided to desensitize Cameron to the commode so he could be potty trained. She made a picture of a stick figure standing next to a toilet to distinguish between standing near the toilet and actually using it, to prevent confusion later. Then she paired that picture with a picture of a reward Cameron liked a lot. She began scheduling time to stand on a fuzzy rug he liked. At first, Mom placed the rug a few feet from the sink. She showed Cameron the pictures, had him stand on the rug, and set a timer for several seconds. She had only the nightlight on and played his favorite music. When the timer signaled, she reinforced him with the reward. Mom gradually moved the rug closer to the toilet and lengthened the time. They completed this routine using the same times she planned to use for habit training, so there were several sessions each day. Within two weeks, Cameron was touching the toilet when shown a picture that cued him. After less than three weeks, he sat on the toilet with no resistance when given the picture cue. Within six weeks he was remaining continent using a habit schedule, pictures and rewards.

Repeated Flushing

When some individuals enter the bathroom, they may repeatedly flush every urinal or toilet in that bathroom. Others may flush one commode over and over. For some, it may be due to not understanding expected behavior in the restroom. For others, the sight of the toilet provides a visual cue to flush. Anxiety or fear regarding the bathroom or toilet can also trigger impulsive flushing.

Teach someone to flush one time after toileting by:

- Using picture cues before entering the bathroom, to direct the person to sit on the commode
- Using preteaching strategies to direct the person to the correct steps for toileting before entering the bathroom
- In the picture sequence for the toileting routine, including pictures that clearly show when and how many times to flush (it may be necessary to place these pictures on the toilet handle as a reminder when the person impulsively reaches to flush).

CASE EXAMPLE

Sarah was being habit trained. She flushed repeatedly whenever she saw the toilet handle. Ms. Weems, her teacher, drew the universal symbol for "no"—a red circle with a slash—on a transparent, two-inch square sheet. She placed this over the toilet handle. She also included a picture symbolizing "one flush" in the picture sequence of the toileting routine, to show her when she could flush. When it was time to flush, Ms. Weems cued Sarah to remove the "no" sign, flush one time, then place the "no" sign back on the handle. Sarah stopped flushing at the wrong times and remembered to flush only once. Replacing the "no" sign on the toilet handle was a fun ritual and it also reminded her that it was not time to flush.

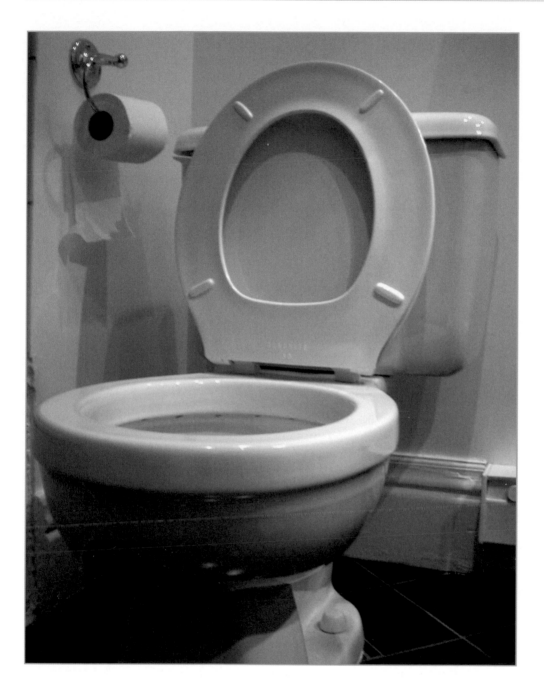

CASE EXAMPLE

Reese used the toilet independently, but flushed over and over. Dad did not want to interfere with his independence, so he had Reese put each picture of his task sequence in an envelope when he finished that step. Once the picture was in the envelope, the task was finished.

Negative Reactions to Taking Away Diapers

Occasionally, someone being toilet trained becomes upset and resists attempts to replace diapers with training pants or underwear. For individuals sensitive to the texture and pressure provided by different types of fabrics or clothing styles, this can be a significant source of discomfort. The satisfying sensations provided by the diaper may come from the tight feel at the legs and waist, the overall pressure of the diaper's snugness against the body, or the feeling of the particular fabric against the skin.

When someone reacts negatively to having diapers replaced with training pants or underpants:

- Place diapers over the underpants and over time gradually cut away or otherwise remove small parts of the diaper, starting with the part that does not provide the greatest amount of satisfying feeling to the person.
- Have him wear underpants instead of diapers for short periods of time daily, gradually increase the number of times per day in underpants, then increase the time frames.
- Use preteaching strategies and reward wearing underpants.

CASE EXAMPLE

Lauren tantrumed when Mom put underpants on her. She enjoyed the snug, thick feeling of her diapers. Mom decided to put underpants on Lauren and put her diaper on top of the underpants. Lauren did not seem to mind this. Mom slowly began fastening the diapers slightly looser each day, until some days they would fall off. This gradual change did not seem to bother Lauren. She would remove the diaper when it was too loose and became accustomed to the feel of underpants. After two weeks of baggy diapers, she would fuss if Mom tried to put a diaper on her.

CASE EXAMPLE

Matthew was toilet trained but resisted wearing underwear instead of a diaper. Mom used his picture schedule to set times for wearing underwear. She used a timer to signal the end of each time period, so he would not accidentally think that misbehavior had ended underwear time. She also used pictures to show the reward he would earn for wearing underwear with no tantrums until the timer signaled the time was finished.

Failure to Urinate in the Toilet

One of the greatest challenges when toilet training someone is to motivate the person to urinate in the commode. Explaining with words seems to be the most logical approach, but it is often ineffective. The problem may be a result of not understanding expectations, a lack of self-control, or anxiety when placed on the toilet.

CASE EXAMPLE

Margarita was on a toileting schedule. Her teacher, Miss Willis, used picture cues and Margarita completed most of the toileting routine independently. Occasionally, Miss Willis had to point to a picture to remind her what to do next. Miss Willis was frustrated because Margarita sometimes went for days without urinating in the toilet. She complied by sitting on the toilet for one or two minutes, then continued with the remainder of the routine. Usually five or ten minutes later, she wet her clothes. Miss Willis decided to give her a cup of water or juice ten minutes before time to potty. She also put a small radio in the restroom and softly played classical music when Margarita was on the commode. Turning off the music became the signal for her to get off the commode and continue her routine. With this signal in place, Miss Willis was able to increase the time Margarita sat on the toilet, which allowed her to relax enough to urinate. These program changes worked immediately. Margarita was using the commode, keeping her clothes dry, and regularly obtaining small rewards for eliminating in the toilet. Following this, she quickly learned to toilet independently and no longer required assistance, extra fluids, music, or rewards.

When someone does not urinate in the toilet:

- Present a clear picture of the desired behavior, using pictures and teaching stories.
- Increase fluid intake several minutes prior to toileting.
- Preteach by reviewing the pictures and reading the related teaching story immediately before the person is toileted.
- Create a relaxing, calm environment using music, favorite calming toys or materials, soothing light levels, and other techniques that help the person relax.
- Minimize words and distractions, whisper to talk.
- Allow the person to remain on the toilet long enough to calm down and relax.

Failure to Have a Bowel Movement in the Toilet

Prompting the learner to have bowel movements in the commode is a toilet training challenge very similar to motivating someone to urinate in the toilet. This problem may also be related to not understanding expectations, a lack of self-control, or anxiety when placed on the toilet, with interventions being basically the same. However, this task is often more difficult to learn, since fewer opportunities for practice are available.

When teaching someone to defecate in the toilet:

- Present a clear picture of the desired behavior using pictures and teaching stories.
- Provide a regular diet, exercise, and adequate fluids.
- Preteach by reviewing the pictures and reading the related teaching story immediately before the person is toileted.
- Create a relaxing, calm environment using music, favorite calming toys or materials, soothing light levels, and other techniques that help the person relax.
- Minimize words and distractions; whisper to talk.
- Allow the person to remain on the toilet long enough to calm down and relax.

CASE EXAMPLE

Darren was twelve years old and had bladder control, but would not defecate in the toilet. When it was the time of day for him to have a bowel movement, he would complete his toileting routine in five minutes or less, without defecating. Ten to twenty minutes later, he would soil his pants. This upset Darren, but he continued with this behavior. Mom decided to teach him to sit on the toilet for longer periods when it was the usual time of day for him to have a bowel movement. She indicated on his picture schedule when to set the timer for twenty minutes for that particular toileting session. She put some of his favorite books beside the commode. Darren enjoyed this quiet time to look at his favorite books. With the extra time and relaxing activities, he was able to remain on the toilet long enough to have a bowel movement. These techniques gave him the extra support needed to stop soiling his clothes.

CAUTION !!!

If urination or defecation seems to be uncomfortable or difficult, consult a physician.

Urinating Outside of the Toilet Bowl

Aiming urine flow into the toilet bowl can present a challenge for some persons. Urinating outside of the bowl may occur because of distractions, not understanding expectations, or problems with physically maintaining self-control.

Promote urinating into the toilet bowl by:

- Minimizing distractions, including talking
- Closing the bathroom door to avoid outside distractions
- Securing a stable physical position for the person
- Using visual cues to show where to aim urine flow
- Providing teaching stories that describe correct techniques
- Preteaching immediately before toileting
- Providing rewards for keeping urine confined to the bowl
- Calmly having the person clean and disinfect any messes, with assistance provided as needed
- Using picture cues to visually show the reward following urination in the commode and clean-up following any messes

CASE EXAMPLE

Mandy had trouble sitting up straight on the toilet seat. Sometimes she leaned backward to rest her head on the toilet tank, in order to stare at the overhead light. When she did this, urine got on her clothes, the toilet seat, and the floor. Mom began using a nightlight in the bathroom, instead of the overhead light. She put a small footstool under Mandy's feet while she sat on the commode. This provided support and a different focus. She also used pictures to show Mandy that when she urinated in the toilet, she was allowed to play with a small flashlight for two minutes after completing her routine. This provided her with the type of visual stimulation she was trying to access, only she received that sensory stimulation after completing an acceptable behavior—urinating in the toilet. Mom placed the pictures showing "urinate in the toilet" and "play with flashlight" on the wall across from the toilet, where Mandy could see them when she sat up correctly on the seat. Mom used preteaching by showing Mandy the pictures when she first entered the bathroom. When Mandy forgot to sit up straight, Mom reminded her by quietly touching the pictures. Within a few days, Mandy was consistently sitting correctly on the toilet with no more messes.

Smearing Feces

A few individuals smear feces on themselves, bathroom walls, and clothing following a bowel movement. Promptly changing this behavior is critical since it presents a highly offensive problem that also carries significant health risks. The safest and most practical approach is to prevent this from occurring in the first place.

To prevent smearing of feces:

- Include in the toileting routine a picture cue to "wipe"; this provides a clear, visual prompt signaling what to do next.
- Provide toilet paper or wipes that are comfortable and easy to use by that particular individual; wet towelettes or warm, wet washcloths are sometimes preferable to persons who are sensitive or poorly coordinated.
- Provide assistance with wiping if needed.
- Regularly check on the person's progress when they are on the toilet; be quiet and subtle when checking.
- Have the person signal when finished, using a bell or similar object.

Once someone has smeared feces, responses need to include:

- Promptly clean and disinfect all contaminated areas.
- If appropriate for that individual, require the person to assist with cleaning and disinfecting.
- Avoid cleaning and disinfecting the mess in front of the person, unless he is participating in the cleanup— watching someone else restore the contaminated areas might be novel and rewarding.
- Minimize any social interaction or talking during cleanup.
- Avoid lecturing, scolding, punishment, complaining, nagging, or emotional reactions.
- Review the picture sequence for the toileting routine, or a teaching story that shows the correct behavior.
- Plan for preventing future smearing by using picture cues, teaching stories, increased supervision, methods for signaling when finished, preteaching, and rewards for completing toileting routines correctly.

CASE EXAMPLE

Blain was being toilet trained using a habit schedule. Mom used a strip of sequenced picture cues to show him the toileting routine. She had accurately identified the time of day when Blain usually had a bowel movement. When he was toileted at this time, she had him sit on the commode and listen to his favorite music, so he would relax enough to defecate. If Mom stayed in the bathroom, he would not relax enough to finish, so she used the time to complete some tasks. Sometimes twenty minutes would pass before Blain had a bowel movement. When she noticed he was finished, Mom wiped his bottom. When she was not nearby, he would immediately begin rubbing his bottom, getting feces on his hands and everything he touched. He did not notice that she used toilet paper for wiping, since his attention was focused on trying to stand the way she instructed. Mom decided to use pictures and a teaching story to show him how to wipe. She put the paper on his hand and helped him do it himself. As a reminder, she also placed a picture on the wall, where he could see it when he was sitting on the commode, that showed "wipe." Mom made sure the toilet paper was within easy reach. Blain began wiping himself with the paper and stopped making messes.

Resistance to Using Toilet Paper

People who are sensitive to certain textures of fabric or types of touch sensations, may resist using toilet paper. Others may resist wiping with paper if that specific step is not clearly included in the toileting routine. Some individuals may not understand how to use the paper.

If the learner resists using toilet paper to wipe:

- Include a picture cue that clearly shows "wipe with paper" in the toileting routine.
- Provide toilet paper or wipes that are comfortable and easy to use; wet towlettes or warm, wet washcloths are sometimes preferable to persons who are more sensitive.
- Provide assistance with wiping if needed.
- Teach the correct behavior by providing physical guidance as needed, using picture cues that show how, and reading a related teaching story.
- Preteach immediately before toileting.
- Post a picture where it is readily seen by the person who is sitting on the commode, to remind him to wipe.

CASE EXAMPLE

Alicia was very impulsive and active. When she saw something interesting, she stopped what she was doing and moved toward the novel item. She was toilet trained, but usually had an offensive odor that smelled like soiled pants. The other children at school moved away from her when she smelled bad. Her teacher, Mrs. Henderson, became more observant and noticed that Alicia was not wiping thoroughly after bowel movements. Verbal reminders did not result in consistent change. Mrs. Henderson decided to teach Alicia to use a wet towelette or washcloth to clean herself more thoroughly. She added a picture to Alicia's toileting routine that showed "wash with a wet cloth" following a bowel movement. Mrs. Henderson helped Alicia the first few times until she consistently completed this new step correctly. She left the picture cues where Alicia could see them easily. Mrs. Henderson also kept a supply of wet towelettes within easy reach of Alicia when she was in the bathroom. If Alicia smelled bad when she came out of the bathroom, Mrs. Henderson cued her to return and wash with soap and water, providing physical guidance if needed. After returning to the bathroom a few times, Alicia became more proficient with cleaning up. Eventually, she stopped having an offensive smell.

Using too Much Toilet Paper

Once someone has learned to use toilet paper, accessing a reasonable amount of paper can pose a problem. Some people do not use enough and others use too much.

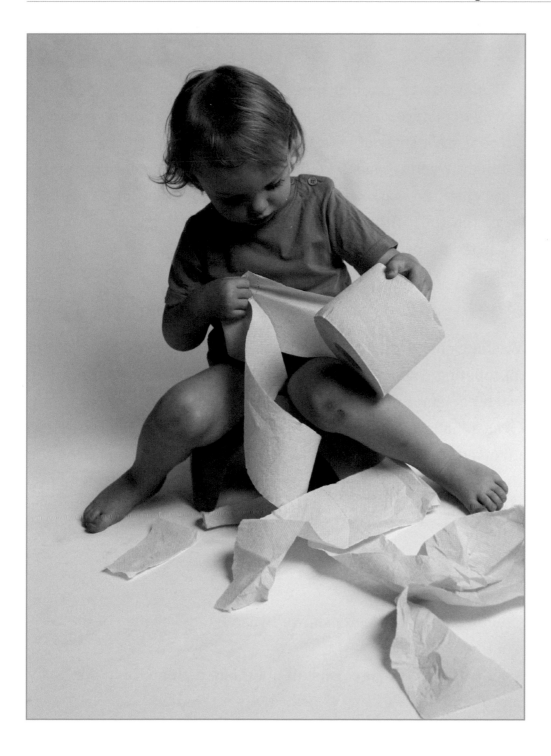

When teaching someone how much toilet paper to use:

* Have him count a specific number of squares of tissue.
* Use visual cues to help determine the right amount.

CASE EXAMPLE

Wendy used too much toilet paper. Since she responded so well to picture cues, Dad placed an obvious mark on the bathroom wall, several inches below the roll of toilet tissue. He taught Wendy to measure the paper by unrolling until the end touched the mark on the wall, then to tear that much paper off the roll. With the help of a visual cue, Wendy was very careful to measure the correct amount of paper.

Resistance to Washing Hands

Washing hands, preferably with soap and water, should be part of all toileting routines. Besides decreasing the risk of illness, handwashing can be a consistent ritual that many people enjoy. Occasionally, individuals resist handwashing or some of the steps involved. This may be due to intolerance for the sensations of touch experienced during the procedure or a limited understanding of expectations.

To teach acceptance of handwashing:

- Include a picture cue that clearly shows "wash hands" as part of the toileting routine.
- Provide soap and towels that consist of materials with textures the person can tolerate.
- Wipe hands with sanitizing cloths if soap and water are completely intolerable.
- Teach the correct behavior by providing physical guidance as needed, using picture cues that show how, and reading a related teaching story.
- Preteach immediately before toileting.
- Follow handwashing with lotion, powder, or other reward.

CASE EXAMPLE

Patrick did not like the feel of soap. He was combative when made to wash his hands after toileting. Mom substituted liquid soap for the usual bar soap. Patrick enjoyed working the squirt mechanism on the soap holder. He tolerated the liquid soap better than the jelly-like feel the bar soap had at times. Since he liked the squirt bottle so much, Mom let Patrick use one squirt of hand lotion as a reward, after he washed his hands with soap. Handwashing was not a problem anymore.

Needing Frequent Cues to Complete Routines

When frequent verbal reminders are repeatedly needed to complete parts of toileting routines, provide the learner with interventions that will enable him to complete these tasks more independently.

To reduce the number of verbal reminders needed:

- Replace repeated verbal prompts with clear visual cues.
- Read teaching stories that describe the task being done.

CASE EXAMPLE

Kendrick's teacher, Mr. Warren, had to remind him to flush the toilet and turn the water off every time Kendrick used the bathroom. Mr. Warren decided to put pictures showing "flush" and "water faucet" on the inside of the restroom door, at Kendrick's eye level to remind him to complete these two tasks. Kendrick completed these tasks consistently, without any more verbal reminders from Mr. Warren.

Resistance to Using Unfamiliar Toileting Facilities

Accessing toileting facilities that are in unfamiliar places, are very large, have many people, or have unusual furnishings can be frightening for someone who has autism. The anxiety created by these differences may interfere with completing toileting routines.

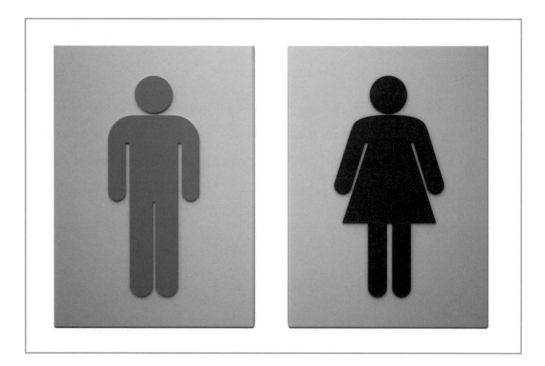

When accessing unfamiliar restroom facilities,
carry a survival kit with familiar visual cues and
calming objects such as wet towelettes or ear plugs.

CASE EXAMPLE

Mom never knew how Lionel was going to react when he used a restroom in an unfamiliar place. Sometimes he was curious and cooperative. Other times he reacted with agitation and tantrums. She could not determine what would upset him. She started carrying the picture sequence he used at home for toileting. When she remembered to show it to him before they entered an unfamiliar restroom, he was cooperative, with no problems. If he started acting anxious, she simply directed his attention back to the pictures and he would complete his toileting routine. She did not need to determine what factors made him resistant under some circumstances, since she already discovered a solution to the problem.

Toilet Trained at Home, but Not at School

Some children are easier to toilet train in the very familiar environment of home. School naturally involves greater or different performance demands than home does, and may create more anxiety, stimulation, and distractions. For some children, the home may provide an environment more conducive to learning to use the toilet.

When a child is toilet trained at home but not at school:

- Parents and teachers need to share information.
- Analyze what factors are in place at home that result in successfully using the toilet.
- Duplicate those factors at school, using the same materials, toileting schedule, and cuing process.
- Continue regular communication between home and school.

CASE EXAMPLE

Ms. Hernandez had tried unsuccessfully for several months to toilet train Hector at school. His mother said he was toilet trained at home. Ms. Hernandez met with Mom to discover what motivated Hector to follow a toileting routine at home. Mom said he had a favorite toy he held while on the commode. She started sending the toy to school with him. Ms. Hernandez paired a picture cue with the toy. Hector used the toilet at school and eventually responded to the picture without the toy. This solution was a result of the teacher and parent working together.

Toilet Trained at School, but Not at Home

Some children respond more favorably to the school environment when learning toileting routines. School settings are often more conducive to following schedules consistently and providing the visual structures needed for learning abstract concepts.

When a child is toilet trained at school, but not at home:

- Wait until effective strategies are developed and the child is having some success with the program before beginning home training.
- Identify the strategies that are effective and duplicate those at home, using the same materials, toileting schedule, routines, and cueing process with appropriate modifications as needed to create a program that is reasonable for the home environment.
- Target toilet training as one of the goals for in-home training and parent training sessions.
- Continue regular communication between school and home.

CASE EXAMPLE

Mrs. Jones was potty training Sammy at school. She had to make a few adjustments to his toileting schedule and the picture cues she was using. Finding the best way to seat him on the toilet also involved some trial and error. Mom was eager to begin potty training Sammy at home, but Mrs. Jones encouraged her to wait until she discovered which approaches worked best, to avoid the burden of making numerous changes at home. She waited until Sammy was eliminating on the toilet on most days, seldom wetting or soiling his clothes, before she taught his routine to Mom. When she shared the approaches with Mom, Mrs. Jones gave her copies of the picture cues being used, helped her develop a toileting schedule that was workable at home, and explained the actual step-by-step procedures for completing his routine. Then she and Sammy completed the routine while Mom watched. They continued to talk or write short notes to each other to answer questions, send progress reports, or share relevant information. The teacher and parent worked together to help Sammy learn to apply his new toileting skills to other situations outside of school. Mrs. Jones' approach made this task easier for Mom, who could have been easily overwhelmed by trying to carry out a program that was still changing.

Regression or Setbacks

Occasionally a person who is being toilet trained or who already independently accesses toileting facilities may begin wetting or soiling clothing or bedding more frequently than usual. These setbacks can be frustrating and upsetting for care providers and the individual who is regressing.

Some people may experience regression or setbacks regarding toileting habits in response to:

- Illness, disease, accident, or significant physical influences
- Medication changes
- Changes in food or fluid consumption
- Changes in sleep patterns
- Significant changes in daily routines
- Changes in family structure or home environment
- Changes regarding school, classmates, assigned classes, performance demands, or significant persons in the school environment
- Increased levels of stress or anxiety

When someone experiences regression or setbacks regarding toileting behavior:

- Identify the cause by exploring changes that occurred immediately prior to the regression.
- Discuss any relevant physical issues with a physician.
- Minimize the impact of any identified causes by using picture cues, teaching stories, comforting objects, increased rest and relaxation breaks, and increased time with preferred persons.
- Return to using the strategies that resulted in success when the person was being trained, including cues, supportive materials, stories, environmental changes, preferred objects, relaxation activities, and survival kits.

CAUTION !!!

Avoid responding with anger, disappointment, or other negative emotions when someone experiences toileting setbacks. This only compounds the problem. Calmly return to effective training strategies.

CASE EXAMPLE

Marcus and his family were very happy in their new house. However, Marcus began wetting and soiling his clothes in the daytime and wetting the bed at night. His parents were frustrated and perplexed since he had been toilet trained more than a year ago. They decided to take out the old items they used to toilet train him. They found his daily picture schedule that included toileting times, the sequenced pictures for his toileting routine, and the related teaching story. Marcus began following the same routines as when he was first learning to use the toilet. He soon was back on schedule with no problems, so his parents put away the pictures, schedule, and teaching story. These old familiar items provided the comfort and support he needed in a time of change.

For some individuals toilet training is achieved easily with the use of a few effective strategies. Others may require a lengthy training period with numerous techniques employed. No matter how challenging the task, the successful investment of our time and effort spent on toilet training will help someone with autism become more independent and provide greater opportunity for positive experiences in home, school and the community.

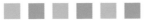

APPENDIX

Data Collection Form for Toilet Training
An Example Social Story—Using the Toilet
Glossary
Resources

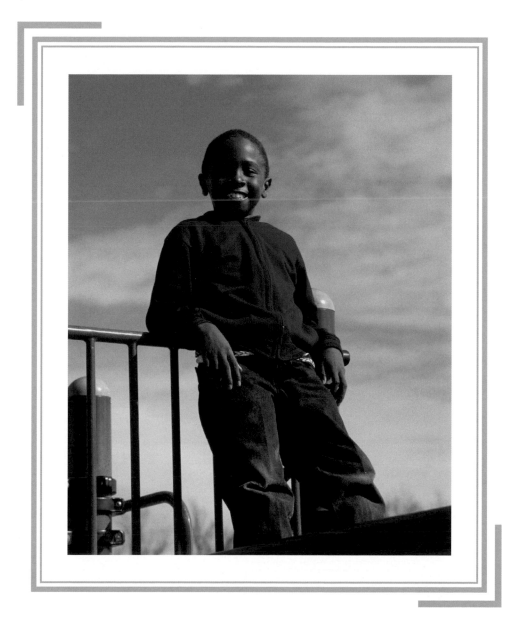

CHART FOR RECORDING OBSERVATIONS OF ELIMINATION TIMES AND RESPONSES.

INSTRUCTIONS: Enter the dates in the heading boxes, using month/day format. In the correct date column, next to the time the person eliminates in clothing (accident) or toilet, indicate observations, using the key below.

KEY: U = Urinated in toilet   B = Bowel movement in toilet

UX = Urinated (accident)   BX = Bowel movement (accident)

Time									
7:00									
7:30									
8:00									
8:30									
9:00									
9:30									
10:00									
10:30									
11:00									
11:30									
12:00									
12:30									
1:00									
1:30									
2:00									
2:30									
3:00									
3:30									
4:00									
4:30									
5:00									
5:30									
6:00									
6:30									
7:00									
7:30									
8:00									
8:30									
9:00									

Comments: _____

_____

Example of a Social Story Related to Toileting

Written on the following page is an example of a story that can be used to teach someone the steps involved when using the toilet. Ideally, stories such as this should be read to the person on a daily basis and immediately before he uses the toilet. The story can be even more effective when illustrated with drawings or pictures, especially when the pictures are the same ones as used to provide visual cues for completing the toileting routine. The story should be arranged so that each step in the routine is on a different page, with only one to three sentences per page. In this example, extra spaces between sections in the story indicate where new pages start. The writing may also be modified by adding the learner's name, so the story is written in a way that describes that person completing the toileting routine correctly. This particular story was written for a child, using the slang words his family spoke when making reference to toileting. Many people may have different preferences regarding the terminology to use in the story. Be sure to use the actual words you say, even if slang words are used, when writing the sentences. Use stories that fit your needs. Different aspects of the toileting routine may present challenges for some learners. Providing a similarly composed story that describes the steps for handwashing may be appropriate for someone who has problems completing the steps for handwashing.

Using the Toilet

Sometimes I have to pee-pee.
I go to the bathroom when I have to pee-pee.

Sometimes I have to poop.
I go to the bathroom when I have to poop.

When I go in the bathroom, I pull my pants down.
I sit on the toilet.

Sometimes I pee-pee in the toilet.
Sometimes I poop in the toilet.

When I am finished going pee-pee and poop, I wipe
my bottom with toilet paper. Sometimes I have to wipe
again. I wipe to make my bottom clean and dry.

After I wipe, I drop the dirty toilet paper in the toilet.
I flush the toilet.

I go to the sink and wash my hands with soap and water.
I dry my hands.

Glossary

Alternative communication system refers to an organized method for communication that uses nonverbal supports such as pictures, picture symbols, or gestures for expressing or receiving information.

Anxiety is a general feeling of uneasiness or mental distress.

Autism is a developmental disability, usually appearing in the first three years of life. It is a neurological disorder involving the brain that usually affects language usage and communication, social interaction, and cognitive processes.

Back-up plan refers to alternate strategies to be implemented if the initial approach is ineffective or not used.

Backward chaining is a strategy in which a skill is broken into smaller steps that are presented and taught in a sequence, starting with the last step first.

Bladder control is the ability to voluntarily restrain urination.

Bowel control is the ability to voluntarily restrain defecation.

Chronological age is the length of time a person has existed as measured by using date of birth.

Comforting sensation is information physically perceived by the body that has a calming affect.

Concrete describes objects, actions, or behaviors that can be physically perceived by the body or directly related to specific or actual objects, actions, or behaviors.

Concrete thinking   refers to thoughts that are directly related to specific or actual objects, actions, or behaviors that can be physically perceived by the body.

Continence or continent   refers to maintaining bladder and bowel control.

Desensitize   is to make someone less sensitive or reactive to particular sources of stimulation or excitement.

Disruptiveness   refers to the degree with which something interrupts or interferes with ongoing activities.

Environmental stimulation   is anything physically perceived by the body that results in a state of increased arousal.

Frustration   refers to the feelings of disappointment experienced when unable to overcome an obstacle.

Habit training   refers to the process in which someone is taught to eliminate on the toilet at specific times of the day, as opposed to accessing the toilet when one is physically aware of the need to eliminate.

Imitation   is mimicking or copying another's actions.

Impulsive   describes unplanned, sudden, spontaneous acts.

Inattentive   refers to concentration and thought being absent or directed toward another point of focus.

Incontinent   describes the inability to restrain or control urination and/or defecation.

Interaction   is the process of mutual exchange between two or more people.

Internet   refers to a computerized communication network that can aid with accessing information from a variety of sources.

Intervention   is the process used to impose changes.

Irrelevant details   describes perceived information that is unimportant or not connected to the topic of focus.

Journal articles   are informative writings in professional publications called journals.

Literal   is the exact, concrete meaning of words, phrases, and sentences.

Literal communication   refers to using the exact, concrete meanings when sharing information with others.

Literal thinking   describes thoughts based upon exact, concrete meanings.

Maladaptive behaviors   are actions that are not suited for, or effective under, the current circumstances.

Mental age   refers to the age level at which a person functions or performs.

Motor planning difficulties   are problems initiating the muscle movements needed to perform a task.

Natural schedule   refers to the use of naturally occurring events to determine preplanned times for toileting.

Noneducational monies   are a relatively small pool of public school funds for items or services deemed not to be necessary for educational benefit. Strict guidelines govern the distribution of these funds.

Noncompliance   is the failure to follow an instruction, demand, or expectation.

Nonverbal behavior   describes actions observed, without considering accompanying words.

Object swap   refers to a system of communication in which representational objects are exchanged for requested objects, activities, or actions as a form of communication.

Offensive hygiene   refers to a level of personal cleanliness that others find unpleasant.

Panic attacks   are episodes of extreme anxiety in which various physical changes occur, such as heart palpitations, shortness of breath, dizziness, trembling, or nausea.

Parent conference   is a meeting between one or more educators and a student's parent(s) to discuss issues related to the student's education.

Physiological factors   are influences created by physical processes in the body.

Picture-based communication   is the use of visual representations of objects, actions, or ideas when sharing information with others.

Picture cues   are visual representations of objects, actions, or ideas used to signal someone to initiate an action or response.

Picture exchange   refers to a communication process that involves exchanging or trading a picture or picture symbol for the object, action, or response it represents.

Picture schedules   are timetables that include preplanned activities represented by visual images.

Picture symbols   are simplistic line drawings used in alternative communication systems that represent objects, actions, or responses.

Positive reinforcers   are any pleasurable actions, objects, or activities that follow a behavior and cause that behavior to increase.

Potty chairs   are freestanding, portable toilets, available in a variety of sizes, materials, and styles.

Potty seats   are supportive devices to be placed on the toilet.

Preteaching   is reminding a person of task steps, expectations, or desired behavior immediately prior to an experience warranting its use.

Regression   is return to a former state of performance.

Reinforcers   are actions, objects, or activities that follow a behavior and cause that behavior to increase. Reinforcers may be positive or negative in nature.

Relaxation break   refers to a period of time devoted to engaging only in activities that have a calming affect.

Respite care   is the provision of a temporary care provider while the permanent care provider is temporarily relieved of caretaking responsibilities.

Reward refers to something, usually with a pleasurable quality, that is given to a person in return for performance.

Rituals are formally repeated patterns of actions.

Role model is someone whom another person observes and mimics.

Routine is a regular course of action, often governed by procedural rules.

Sensitivity to stimulation refers to an extreme reaction in response to physical sensations or changes perceived by the body.

Sensory awareness is the degree of responsiveness to perceived physical sensations.

Sensory input refers to physical sensations perceived by the body.

Sensory issues refer to behavior, performance or other topics of discussion or concern that are related to reactions toward physical sensations or changes perceived by the body.

Sequenced chain of behaviors is a connected series of actions forming a more complex act.

Sequence of steps is a connected series of actions performed in a specific order, to form a more complex task.

Sequential learning refers to acquiring new information by connecting a series of ideas or experiences in a specific order.

Setback is loss of progress made toward a goal.

Siblings refer to brothers and sisters.

Social acceptance is being received and welcomed willingly and gladly by other people.

Social skills training refers to the process of teaching the behaviors needed for social acceptance.

Special education support refers to the assistance available through public school special education programs.

Stimulation   is something that causes or promotes a response.

Stress   refers to physiological changes that occur in response to stimulation or change.

Stress management techniques   are strategies used to decrease the negative impact of stimulation and change.

Support groups   are people with a common interest who meet in an effort to provide for the similarly related needs of one another.

Tactile stimulation   is anything perceived through physical contact that increases arousal.

Tantrums   refer to episodes of unacceptable behaviors that disrupt ongoing activities and may consist of intense actions such as screaming, stomping feet, throwing objects, or aggression.

Toilet training   is a procedure for teaching someone to use the toilet for urination or defecation.

Training pants   are specially designed undergarments to wear during the period of toilet training, in place of diapers. They are made with extra padding in strategic locations for better absorption.

Verbal cue or verbal prompt   is the use of words to stimulate a response.

Verbalization   is oral expression of wants, needs, thoughts, feelings, or ideas using word approximations, words, phrases, or sentences.

Visual cue or visual prompt   is the presentation of a stimulus perceived through the eyes to stimulate a response.

Visual schedule or visually-based schedule   refers to a timetable that includes preplanned activities represented by visual images.

Visual thinkers   describes persons who create visual images in their mind in order to attach meaning to language.

Vocalization   is expression of wants, needs, thoughts, feelings, or ideas consisting of orally produced noises that are not spoken words.

References and Resources

Ando, H. (1977). "Training Autistic Children to Urinate in the Toilet Through Operant Conditioning Techniques." *Journal of Autism and Childhood Schizophrenia*, 7, 151–163.

Ayres, A.J. (1979). *Sensory Integration and the Child*. Los Angeles, CA: Western Psychological Services.

Azrin, N.H., Bugle, C., & O'Brien, F. (1971). "Behavioral Engineering: Two Apparatuses for Toilet Training Retarded Children." *Journal of Applied Behavior Analysis*, 4, 89–99.

Butler, J. (1976). "Toilet Training a Child with Spina Bifida." *Journal of Behavior Therapy and Experimental Psychiatry*, 7, 63–65.

Fouse, B., & Wheeler, M. (1997). *A Treasure Chest of Behavioral Strategies for Individuals with Autism*. Arlington, TX: Future Horizons, Inc.

Foxx, R.M., & Azrin, N.H. (1973). *Toilet Training the Retarded*. Champaign, IL: Research Press.

Frost, L.A., & Bondy, A.S. (1994). PECS. *The Picture Exchange Communication System: Training Manual*. Cherry Hill, NJ: Pyramid Educational Consultants, Inc.

Grandin, T. (1995). *Thinking in Pictures*. New York, NY: Doubleday.

Gray, C. (1993). *The Original Social Story Book*. Arlington, TX: Future Horizons, Inc.

Gray, C. (1994). *The New Social Story Book*. Arlington, TX: Future Horizons, Inc.

Hodgdon, L.A. (1995). *Visual Strategies for Improving Communication*. Troy, MI: QuirkRoberts Publishing.

Individuals with Disabilities Education Act of 1990. Federal Register. 57, (189), September 29, 1992.

Kimbrell, D.L., et al. (1967). "Operation Dry Pants: An Intensive Habit Training Program for Severely and Profoundly Retarded." *Mental Retardation*, 5, 32–36.

Mayer-Johnson Company. *The Picture Communication Symbols Books I, II, and III.* Solana Beach, CA: Mayer-Johnson Company.

Willbarger, P., & Willbarger, J.L. (1991). *Sensory Defensiveness in Children, Age Two to Twelve: An Intervention Guide for Parents and Other Caretakers.* Santa Barbara, CA: Avanti Educational Programs.

Williams, M.S. (1994). *How Does Your Engine Run? A Leader's Guide to the ALERT Program for Self-regulation.* Albuquerque, NM: Therapy Works, Inc.

Yonovitz, A., & Michaels, R. (1977). "Durable, Efficient, and Economical Electronic Toilet Training Devices for Use with Retarded Children." *Behavior Research Methods and Instrumentation*, 9, 356–358.

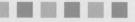

Index

About the Author

Maria Wheeler has spent more than twenty years of her professional life in the fields of Psychology and Special Education, with an emphasis on Neurobehavioral Disorders, Applied Behavior Analysis, and Specific Learning Disabilities. She has held positions in Florida and Texas as a special education classroom teacher, behavior specialist, and director of behavioral services for residential treatment centers serving adults and children with neurobehavioral disorders and developmental disabilities. She currently holds Texas teacher certficates/endorsements in Serious Emotional Disturbance and Autism, Special Education, and Psychology.

Maria works as a private consultant serving various school districts, educational agencies, and families throughout Texas. She is a nationally recognized speaker and trainer in the fields of autism, behavior and learning disorders, and effective discipline. She provides on-site behavior intervention and classroom curriculum consultation for educators of students with autism and other behavior and learning disorders. She also provides on-site coaching for in-home trainers and tutors, parent training, and professional development training. Maria authored the popular book entitled, *Discipline That Works for Inclusive Schools*, published by RealWorld Publications. She co-authored one of the leading manuals on behavior, *A Treasure Chest of Behavioral Strategies for Individuals with Autism*, published by Future Horizons, Inc.

Hay Library
Western Wyoming Community College